the SUNLIGHT SOLUTION

WHY MORE SUN EXPOSURE AND VITAMIN D ARE ESSENTIAL TO YOUR HEALTH

the
SUNLIGHT
SOLUTION

WHY MORE SUN EXPOSURE
AND VITAMIN D
ARE ESSENTIAL
TO YOUR HEALTH

laurie winn carlson

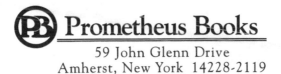
Prometheus Books

59 John Glenn Drive
Amherst, New York 14228-2119

Published 2009 by Prometheus Books

Inquiries should be addressed to
Prometheus Books
59 John Glenn Drive
Amherst, New York 14228–2119
VOICE: 716–691–0133, ext. 210
FAX: 716–691–0137
WWW.PROMETHEUSBOOKS.COM

13 12 11 10 09   5 4 3 2 1

Library of Congress Cataloging-in-Publication Data

Carlson, Laurie W., 1952–
    The sunlight solution : why more sun exposure and vitamin D are essential to your
health / by Laurie Winn Carlson
        p. cm.
    Includes bibliographical references and index.
    ISBN 978–1–59102–701–0 (pbk. : alk paper)
    1. Sunlight. 2. Vitamin D Deficiency—complications. 3. Vitamin D Deficiency—his-
tory. 4. Vitamin D Deficiency—prevention and control. I. Title

QP82.2.L5C37 2009
612.3'99—dc22

                                                                        2008054563

Printed in the United States on acid-free paper

This book is for Brian and Tyler, who know firsthand the value of sunlight. And for Anaxagoras, the Greek philosopher, who ended his promising career in 500 BCE by pointing out that the sun was a fiery rock and not God.

CONTENTS

ACKNOWLEDGMENTS

Writing about a topic as expansive as sunlight meant contacting a variety of people in far-flung fields of study. I am very grateful for everyone who responded to e-mails, letters, phone calls, and personal conversations: William B. Grant at the Sunlight, Nutrition, and Health Research Center in San Francisco; Dr. Reinhold Vieth at Mount Sinai Hospital in Toronto; Dr. George Studzinski at New Jersey Medical School and colleagues Ela Gocek and Dr. David Hislop; Dr. Robert P. Heaney at Creighton University; Professor Graham Farquhar at Australian National University; Dr. John Jacob Cannell at the Vitamin D Council; and Dr. Dale W. Griffin at the US Geological Survey were all very helpful. Thanks to Robert Darby, Jennifer Anne Hamilton, Steven Arrowsmith of the Worldwide Fistula Fund; Bill Obermeyer at Consumerlab.com; Stacy Davis at the National Multiple Sclerosis Society/Inland Northwest Chapter; Mary Ann Parr, Consumer Relations, Organic Valley/CROPP Cooperative; Mike Nygaard at West Farm Foods; Carol Haggans at the Office of Dietary Supplements of the National Institutes of Health; Paul Stamets at Fungi Perfecti; Mary Beth Huber of Osteogenesis Imperfecta Foundation; Dr. Matt Layton at Spokane Mental Health; Greg Hartung of Wilcox Farms; Steve and Kate Shay at Oregon State University; Nancy Giese at St. Aloysius Elementary School; nutritionist Krispin Sullivan; Todd Wylie, OD; and Charles Bowman, as well as many others who gave me information when I wasn't sure what questions I should even be asking. The book would not be possible without the astute and patient guidance of several others, especially Doreen Valentine, Audra Wolfe, Joe Gramlich, and Chris Kramer, whose insights and advice improved the manuscript immensely. Steven L. Mitchell at Prometheus Books recognized my mission with the book and helped me find an audience. I appreciate him and his helpful insights and enthusiasm for the project. Thanks also to the young women at the local tanning salon, who don't snicker each week when I arrive to use a tanning bed for only a few minutes; I'm surely their only regular customer who doesn't want to actually tan. They did give me valuable advice before hitting the beds: "At your age, I'd cover my face with a towel." Good point.

Introduction

THE SUNSHINE SOLUTION

The idea that sunlight is essential to health may come as a surprise—at least it did to me. Plants need it, yes, but people? Our highly sophisticated, information-based indoor culture, which I am completely embedded in as a writer in the Pacific Northwest, has pretty much ignored our relationship to the sun. We eat natural foods, appreciate nature, and work to preserve the environment, yet we rarely leave our workplaces, homes, or automobiles. Sunlight—something seemingly commonplace yet actually absent from many of our daily lives—is crucial to human life, but we ignore it as part of our environment.

Today, those in the medical field look to molecular biologists for new interventions to optimize health, but there are some old-fashioned ideas that shouldn't be overlooked. Sunlight is what we're missing; like the bean plant experiment in the second-grade classroom, if we don't get enough sunlight, we droop and die. Plants need sunlight for photosynthesis—we understand that process—but our own skin cells need to take in sunlight, too, in a process that's only just becoming understood.

I'm not a physician; I am a historian. I look at broad patterns of change and how humans relate to those changes. Trends in health, medicine, and disease, traced from antiquity to the present, are fascinating. Many of the ideas from the past—such as bloodletting—are outmoded today, but they remind us how far medicine and science have come. Students enjoy digging into the past, and lots of intriguing questions and issues always come up. So I wasn't surprised when a college student in my history of medicine class remarked about how rickets, a disease we think of as connected to the nineteenth century, might be something to worry about today. We had been discussing a nineteenth-century image of young boys employed as coal miners and another of girls working in textile factories, their skeletons shrunken, their eyes listless and glazed over. Lack of sunlight—in the days before we really understood nutrition and healthcare—doomed such children, who seldom went outdoors. Little girls grew to adulthood with stunted pelvic bones due to childhood rickets, making normal births impossible and leading to painful death in childbirth if they could not afford surgical deliveries.

Rickets as a childhood ailment has been around a long time and was written about in 1650 by Francis Glisson, a medical professor at Cambridge University. He was first to give a clinical description of the bone disorder and termed it rickets, explaining the name came from the Old English word *wrikken*, which means to bend or twist.

Rickets is a deficiency disease in which young growing bones become spongy and soft. Children develop bowed legs or knock-knees and their head and torso often appear out of proportion to their short legs. I remember those health and nutrition textbooks that always included an image of a misshapen youngster, standing naked before the camera. Their diet was only part of the cause. Children's lives in the nineteenth century (and in the twentieth century before compulsory education laws) were often filled with long work days spent toiling in factories or mine shafts. They ate poorly, were overworked, and needed rest and fresh air. They lived in smoky, polluted cities, without parks or playgrounds. Thankfully, those dismal lives are relics of the past as advances in science, technology, and social policy have moved ahead.

Like other health problems of the nineteenth century, rickets was "cured" by scientific discovery and modern healthcare. Wasn't it? My student insisted that such a conclusion might not be true. Didn't children today (and college students like her peers) spend the majority of their time indoors? How were their lives different—if you were looking at the amount of time average students spend outdoors—compared to the child laborers in dim mines and factories of the past? she insisted. "Television and computers," she argued. "They keep us tethered inside."

"Air-conditioning, too," a classmate added. The class looked at me expectantly.

Well, what *were* the facts? I dug through a few current family medical guides—nothing there. Going to the Internet, I wasn't sure what to look for, but I quickly found plenty of research to suggest my student was correct. Indeed, there were a few researchers who warned of a return to the past. There were sporadic cases of rickets reported across the country. Children were showing up in hospitals with the sunlight deficiency disease again, even in the southern United States, where one expects people would receive plenty of sunshine. Some researchers went so far as to warn of an unrecognized modern epidemic of rickets.

VITAMIN D, THE "SUNSHINE VITAMIN"

The sun's action on our body creates vitamin D—the "sunshine" vitamin. It isn't a true vitamin, however, but a hormone created in the body through a metabolic process involving the intestines, liver, kidneys, and blood, sparked by ultraviolet (UV) light rays on skin cells. The body's creation of vitamin D is a complicated process so it's no surprise that the process isn't completely understood and has only been investigated in recent years—almost a century after it was identified as an essential nutrient. One might say that vitamin D from sunlight is the ultimate environmental link connecting us to the cosmos. Without it, we fade and ultimately die. Yet too much UV radiation is a killer, as any dermatologist or skin cancer specialist can tell you. Fine-tuning our relationship with the sun is essential and scientists are only just beginning to recognize the many and varied ways our body depends upon UV light.

When we think about all the hours we spend indoors, it seems quite possible that we would experience sunlight deficiency. It can only be confirmed by testing blood levels of vitamin D, such as the clinical signs of its deficiency. While large numbers of children aren't suffering from full-blown rickets today, a less serious level of deficiency may unknowingly affect hundreds of thousands of youngsters. Indeed, a vitamin D deficiency is hard to identify until the individual is extremely debilitated. Inadequate bone growth has been the most common indicator and that takes years to recognize. Some of the more vague symptoms of vitamin D deficiency include:

- diarrhea
- insomnia
- leg cramps
- nervousness
- nonspecific back pain
- periodontal disease
- pigeon chest (discussed below)
- poor teeth

- slowed growth
- vision problems

As I researched to better discuss the issue with my students, the phrase "pigeon chest," referring to a malformation of the ribs and sternum so that it juts out on the child's chest, riveted my attention. This array of problems, and in particular the reference to a misshapen rib formation, matched a list of problems one of my grandsons had been experiencing. Several family members had remarked on the way Brian's ribs and sternum seemed to jut out, but no one had been able to figure it out. And the list of other symptoms? He had them all.

Could it be he was deficient in vitamin D? I'd never heard of anyone being deficient in vitamin D, at least in this century. It seemed to be one of those innocuous staples of life you just take for granted, like water. Besides, I remembered from home economics nutrition classes years ago that you could get too much vitamin D, actually endangering your health. Vitamin D is like vitamin A, a fat-soluble vitamin that is stored in the body, so ingesting too much can be toxic.[1]

I had not given any thought to vitamin D or its connection to sunlight when I first began trying to figure out and remedy my grandson's health problems. Between the ages of three and seven years, Brian experienced an array of health problems that, while not life threatening, were worrisome. They were the sort of things a grandmother notices—and worries about—but they didn't seem to connect to any recognizable syndrome. His front teeth appeared to be disintegrating, wearing away at the edges. Dentists told his mother he was obviously grinding his teeth at night. But these were front teeth, not molars, which had already decayed and been replaced with crowns. Further, Brian slept with his mouth open because his tonsils were so enlarged he had a hard time breathing at night. His pediatrician advised a wait-and-see approach to treating his condition with a tonsillectomy. In kindergarten, a vision screening sent him to an optometrist for glasses, but eyeglasses don't ring warning bells for a systemic and chronic health condition. It was his behavior we worried most about. He was clearly saddled with a severe case of attention deficit hyperactive disorder (ADHD). His nervousness and inattentiveness seemed to overshadow everything else, and fortunately medication worked quite well to manage his behavior. Nonetheless, his nighttime insomnia and complaints of leg pain continued. Advice came from all directions: some said he complained because he wanted more attention; others that his leg pain was psychosomatic in order to control the situation; or his insomnia was because he sought soothing music and stories at bedtime. His mother tried filling his room with pleasant, relaxing smells, administering herbal tea to relax him, and playing calming music. I provided stories, massages, and warm milk when he stayed at my house. But he remained an unhappy little boy.

As I said, we never thought of his complaints as life threatening, but they nagged at us. He seemed to have a recurring case of diarrhea. Pediatricians said not to worry; boys have trouble with that sort of thing. More time, they said. Don't rush it.

While he was charming and sweet and clever as could be, the situation was not optimal for either his development or his success in school. When he failed to grow very much, we really worried. That's when I began pushing milk, something he had not been getting enough of. His preschool, school lunch, and after-school programs all offered milk to the children, but no one could ensure each child actually drank it. At one program, the children who didn't want to drink their milk were told to put the unopened cartons in a separate box for the homeless shelter. He refused to drink it at home; he preferred juice, and, like many kids today, soda pop was never out of reach.

But there was still cheese—if he wouldn't drink milk, cheese sticks seemed a great solution. They were full of protein and calcium, easy to eat, and he liked them. So cheese sticks, cottage cheese, yogurt, and ice cream became part of his diet. Calcium-fortified orange juice seemed like a godsend for kids who resisted milk; it promised to deliver ample amounts of calcium. We didn't realize it, but we were only getting it half right. In order for the body to process calcium, it needs to have ample amounts of vitamin D stored in the cells. One without the other is practically worthless.[2]

At the time, I was unaware that vitamin D levels could be tested and my suggestion to his pediatrician that he might not have enough vitamin D was ignored. In a moment of serendipity, I noticed an advertisement for chewable vitamin D and calcium supplements and wondered if they might be the answer. Supplemental chews had the advantage of being kid friendly (they are similar to caramel candy) and it's easy to track their intake. Once he began consuming adequate amounts of vitamin D along with calcium in supplements, he made a remarkable recovery. It took many months, but eventually his new teeth grew in to replace his disintegrating baby teeth and he began behaving more calmly. He slept better, his leg pains disappeared, and he even had a sudden two-inch growth spurt. That there was a connection between his improving health and development and the nutritional supplements seemed apparent. Finding the essential nutrient that was missing, something so inexpensive and readily available as vitamin D, was a stroke of luck. As I studied the issue, I realized how vital sunlight and vitamin D are to health and yet how we take them for granted, ignoring how much our lives and health depend on adequate amounts. I decided to write this book because the topic is so essential to preventive health. Because sunlight is taken for granted and cannot be patented, advertisement-driven media give the issue short shrift. My goal in this book is to light the way, so to speak, pointing to research findings and a historical perspective on how significant sunlight is to health; to show how a lack of it, due to modern lifestyles, can cause chronic health problems; and to offer suggestions for developing a strategy for safely getting more sunlight in our lives.

WHAT IS VITAMIN D?

The most surprising thing about vitamin D is that it isn't a vitamin at all. Rather, it is a by-product of a chemical reaction that occurs in our bodies and is triggered by sunlight on our skin. Although biochemists have been studying sunlight's effect within our body for nearly a century, they are only just beginning to understand this complex relationship. In the 1960s it was recognized as a hormone, just like cortisol, testosterone, or progesterone.

When ultraviolet rays from the sun are absorbed by the skin, they activate a derivative of cholesterol, 7-dehydrocholesterol, which is slowly changed to vitamin D_3. The bloodstream carries it to the liver, where it's metabolized to create $25(OH)D_3$. From there, $25(OH)D_3$ moves through the bloodstream to the kidneys, where it is activated as two different vitamin D substances: 1a, 25 $(OH)_2D_3$ and 24R, 25 $(OH)_2D_3$, which are transported to specific organs in the body. From that point, it becomes a complex process, taking place in the skin, the bloodstream, the liver, and the kidneys, before vitamin D moves to the teeth, bones, intestines, muscles (including the heart), and elsewhere. The movement of vitamin D to the various parts of the body that need it is controlled by a hormonal system controlled by the kidneys. When levels of vitamin D in the bloodstream are low, more is produced by the kidney and released into the bloodstream, and vice versa.

In the bloodstream, vitamin D ensures that adequate amounts of the minerals calcium and phosphate are available for bone and tissue health. If adequate amounts aren't available over an extended period of time because there either isn't enough vitamin D or enough of the minerals, then bones and tissues deteriorate and children develop rickets or adults develop osteomalacia, or soft bones. Vitamin D is so powerful that when calcium levels in the bloodstream are low, due to inadequate dietary intake, it will pull calcium from the bones and teeth to raise the blood calcium concentrations. That means calcium levels in someone with an inadequate intake of calcium may *appear* normal when blood calcium levels are tested, but it's only because the calcium is coming from the skeleton, and not the diet. Vitamin D hormone and parathyroid hormone control calcium levels to maintain the body's needs. Normally, dietary sources of calcium (e.g., milk products, vegetables such as broccoli) fill the body's needs first; the internal stores of calcium in bones and teeth are tapped last.

If the body stores too much vitamin D, that can be a problem as well because excess vitamin D suppresses T cell–mediated immune functions, actually suppressing the immune system. T cells are white blood cells that recognize and destroy invaders such as viruses. New findings show that reliance on chemical forms of vitamin D_3 (rather than natural sunlight) found in supplements can actually inhibit the body's immune system, making us more susceptible to infection.[3]

Vitamin D_3, cholecalciferol, is formed in human and animal skin and can also be metabolized from the foods we eat. A similar form, vitamin D_2, is created in certain plants by UV irradiation. Some examples of naturally occurring D_2 are plankton, mushrooms, and ergot. Humans and animals can either make vitamin D from exposure to UV light or from eating sources of D_3 or D_2, such as cod liver oil or mushrooms. Because vitamin D can be absorbed through the digestive system, we tend to think of it inaccurately as a nutrient. Hector F. DeLuca, biochemist at University of Wisconsin–Madison, notes, "We must move away from the concept that vitamin D is a vitamin." It's actually a prohormone that converts to a hormone within the body, and there are very few natural-occurring food sources that contain it in significant levels.[4]

While this seems a simple explanation of physiology, health professionals are not in agreement about how much sunlight our bodies need, or indeed if they should receive much at all. In fact, today the lines are drawn between advocates of sunlight for health and those who warn everyone to stay out of direct sunlight completely to prevent skin cancer and aging. The federal government and medical associations have solidly come out against sunlight exposure, advocating chemical sunscreens and sun avoidance as ways to avoid developing skin cancer. With concerns about the earth's natural UV filter, the ozone layer, being eroded through our use of chlorofluorocarbons (CFCs) and other chemicals, it is responsible to alert the public to the dangerous side of UV exposure. But more important, in an effort to safeguard against one set of health concerns, we cannot neglect others. There are benefits to sunlight, as this book aims to show. Advocates of a sunlight solution form a growing group and their concerns are being acknowledged.

Sunshine? Or shadow? Which is optimal? Can we expose our bodies to enough sunlight to develop healthy stores of vitamin D without also increasing our chances of getting cancerous skin tumors? By avoiding sunlight and living indoor lives are we incurring higher risks perhaps for a bevy of worse conditions? Moderation is key, as well as an understanding of how and when sunlight is most optimal to our health. It's a serious argument, and lives really are on the line.

Vitamin D—the science, the politics, and the need for research—is an intriguing topic of global proportions. The sun, our work-a-day lives under artificial lighting, and the chemistry within our bodies are only part of the story. Our gender and age, where we live and how we live, whether at higher latitudes or under artificial lighting, as well as our diet affect our level of vitamin D, and ultimately our health.

Chapter One

SUN CULTURE BEGINS

Early human societies recognized the sun's power and importance and developed rituals and myths to connect them to what was clearly the dominant life giver on earth. No single force affected life as much as the daily rising and setting of the sun, a relationship that shaped how early people lived and thought. Joy and reverence for sunrise—as well as fear of darkness—evolved into rites led by priests and priestesses who could speak with the sun god or a pantheon of sun-related deities, ensuring continued sunlight.

The realization that without sunlight life on earth would disappear was recognized long before the scientific understanding of photosynthesis. While sunlight's biological actions weren't understood, its significance to life and health was central to early civilizations that believed the sun was either the source of life or the first entity created by a higher being. Life revolved around the sun, so the fear that something might suddenly stop its daily appearance became a powerful motivating force in life and culture. Origin myths often explain the world as steeped in darkness then suddenly lit by the appearance of the sun. In many legends, the end of the world would follow the disappearance of the sun, something to be prevented at all costs.

Clearly, the sun could grant life with its warmth or take it away by disappearing, yet it remained a steady and cyclical power, a condition people attributed to their own efforts through prayer, dance, or even the extreme of human sacrifice. Cultures revered the sun in some way, but how they expressed this and the imagined sun god's character (whether compassionate and just, or cruel and punitive) varied greatly. Interpretations as well as people's behavior regarding the sun were defined by culture as well as by latitude and environment. Because those most dependent upon sunlight, such as agricultural societies and those in the far north, regarded the sun as extremely powerful in daily life, they often resorted to extremes in behavior to please or appease the sun.

People living in cloudless areas with plentiful sunshine who relied on the sea rather than on agriculture for survival could regard the sun with less worry and more joy.

It was natural to link the powerful yet mysterious force of sunlight to the otherworld. How else were they to explain such a phenomenon that seemed alive and omniscient, with strength and cunning unfathomable to the people who depended upon it? As if by magic, it appeared on one side of the world and disappeared over the edge of the opposite side, leaving only darkness in its wake. The need for sunlight to illuminate life was essential because the darkness of night was overwhelming. Today, we rarely think of it unless we're stranded on a remote road without a flashlight, but without electricity at night we're as frightened and helpless as those long ago who heralded the sunrise because it wiped away the darkness.

Day and night were the most important rhythms in daily life, followed by the seasonal changes brought about by the sun's changing position in the sky. The sun's activity followed patterns but was never static and not to be taken for granted. The most important people in sun-worshiping civilizations were those who monitored the sun's activity—the astrologers and calendar keepers—because appeasing the sun required prayer, sacrifice, and ceremonies by everyone in the society. People felt compelled to interfere when the sun seemed to disappear or hide away, such as the elongated nights of winter. Desperately dependent on sunlight, they developed ceremonies to entice the sun to come out of hiding. A Japanese myth in which the sun hides in a cave and humans have to figure out how to lure it out is similar to other symbolic explanations for the sun's cyclical disappearance and reappearance. Trees decorated with shiny objects, prayers, dancing, and lighted fires were used to tempt the sun's curiosity so it would peek out again. Gaining favor with the sun ensured fertility, health, food, and happiness. On the other hand, the sun was an unforgiving god, one that shouldn't be taken for granted. Drought punished everyone and was seen as the sun god's displeasure with the people. Appeasing the sun became a valuable tool in social control and group stability, and individuals needed to behave by common norms for the good of the community. After all, the omniscient sun was overhead, watching everyone.

The seasonal variation in length of day and position of the sun had a profound effect on plants, animals, and humans. Lying low in the sky all winter, then moving directly overhead in summer, the sun's warmth and light changed considerably in higher latitudes. Agriculture relied on a complex understanding of the sun and seasons, requiring the development of calendars, solar festivals, and elaborate efforts to keep track of the sun. This being no simple matter, sites like England's Stonehenge were constructed as huge solar-measuring devices. People paid a great deal of attention to the sun's strength and position in the sky, giving it a variety of names depending upon the time of day or season. The spring sun was most appreciated because it launched the year into growth and vigor once more after a winter sun of reduced strength and presence.[1]

THE SUN IN MYTHOLOGY AND WORLD RELIGIONS

Various interpretations of the sun's actions tried to explain its relationship to the natural world. The "solar myth" that was common in many cultures explained the sun rising up in the morning as a symbolic birth and dropping over the horizon at night as a death, often blamed on being swallowed by a monster. The daily battle between darkness and light was central to humanity's existence, therefore playing a prominent role in religion and cultural mythology. The seasonal sun was also given its place in myths of many cultures, which often described the sun as a baby born daily or seasonally; or a sun child that grew to take on monsters of the night. The sun could be a brilliant or a gloomy god, a friend or an enemy.

While the sun played a prominent role in creation tales, other stories evolved to explain culture and the human condition. Sun god narratives follow a birth, growth, death, and reincarnation pattern, replicating the sun's daily rising, disappearance, and reemergence. In most tales, the sun is a lone individual, male or female, who goes off on a mysterious and dangerous journey to the unknown world of darkness and returns triumphant or at least wiser. Mythic tales of travel to far-off unknown lands emerge from people's curiosity about where the sun went when it vanished from sight every evening. They parallel the Hero's Journey pattern in literature and myth, described by Joseph Campbell. Sun worship led to the emergence of the hero figure, exemplified well by Apollo, the Greek sun god.[2]

Sun myths also helped decipher the workings of the natural world. Nocturnal animals, like owls and bats, are explained as creatures that failed to heed the dictates of proper behavior and were ultimately banished to a dark world.

Cultures such as the Incas of Peru attributed their success to accepting and following the dictates of a larger authority, the sun. Believing their location in a fertile valley of the Andes was due to advice from the sun, they thought other cultures failed to match their achievements because they refused to obey authority.

Mythology created a way to interpret and respect the sun's centrality to life, but it remained distant, unapproachable, and nonhuman. Storytelling simply could not soften the fierceness of the sun; it remained impossible to look at directly and could never be considered mundane. Too much sun creates drought, sunstroke, and sunburn, and results in crop failures, famine, or death. Many tales describe scorching and burning in the flaming heat of a capricious or vindictive sun, such as the Greek tale of Icarus, whose waxen wings melted when he flew too close to the sun's heat. Sun gods could be warm and nurturing—welcomed in the springtime—or scorching and in need of appeasement. Understanding the sun's complex behavior was no simple task and many in the ranks of early priests and astronomers spent their lives charting the sun's movement across the sky, timing its appearance and disappearance and establishing patterns of behavior to optimize its warmth.

Many ancient cultures distinguished between the various rays of the sun, from the brilliant to the gloomy. Just as we note the axiom that Inuit people have many words to represent the many varieties of snow in their world, ancient people had an intense connection to sunlight and its various forms and strengths. Today, we might simply say cloudy or clear and let it go at that. Egyptians separated the sun into entities: the light separate from heat; the orb separate from its rays. Each represented a deity in a polytheistic sun religion.

Greek lore was shaped around the sun: gods threw disks, grabbed thunderbolts, and stayed on mountaintops, close to the sun. The colossal statue at Rhodes was a monument to the sun god Helios. The sun deities and their Greek followers fought the ultimate hell: banishment into total darkness in the form of Hades. The Romans picked up where the Greeks left off, expanding and polishing the sun-themed mythology. Apollo's chariot, whose wheel was the sun, raced across the sky each day, pulled by four horses representing the four types of sunlight: the rising reddish rays; midmorning sun, which is clear; noonday sun in its strength and glory; and the setting sun, which was said to kiss the earth.

The Greeks' panoply of sun-related deities influenced the Romans, who incorporated sun worship ideology into their daily lives, too. Their lives were spent indoors more than the Greeks, but access to sunlight shaped their technology, laws, and customs. In the first century CE, Romans invented window glass to let light inside buildings; pieces almost two inches wide and two feet long have been found in ancient ruins. Wealthy Romans in the imperial period had glazed windows in their homes and Roman gardeners even grew vegetables during winter in glass greenhouses. They also studied passive solar design for buildings and utilized the sun's light and warmth as much as possible, such as building public baths with windows on the south-facing side to let in maximum sunlight. Legislated "sun rights" protected access to sunlight, making it a civil offense for anyone to obstruct someone else's access to sunlight exposure, par-ticularly for buildings that required solar energy for heating and lighting.[3]

Using the sun's light and energy was practical: it provided free energy, acted as a bactericide, fungicide, and cleansing agent. Ultraviolet rays destroy microbes, which would have kept the baths healthier. Ironically, the Romans manipulated the sun so they could enjoy its benefits while staying indoors— behavior that evolved as a mark of social and economic status. Rather than sit outdoors under the natural sun rays like the Egyptians, privileged Romans moved inside, establishing a divide between those who labored under the sun (and tanned), and those who did not have to labor with their hands and bodies. Upper-class Roman women stayed indoors and out of sunlight, applying cos-metics to give them a pale complexion. Their children remained indoors, too, garnering the first recorded cases of childhood rickets. So, in this culture, being tan equaled being a mere laborer or even a slave. Not showing signs of being in the sun was a form of elitism or of high social standing. In much the same way, being obese or heavy was viewed as a sign of wealth.

In 100 CE, Soranus, a Roman physician, wrote *Diseases of Women*, including a chapter on "Why the Majority of Roman Children Are Distorted," which he attributed to their mothers allowing them to sit on cold stone floors. Roman mothers tried to prevent such distortions by wrapping infants tightly in swaddling clothes for their first year, so their bones would grow straight. Tight swaddling clothes remained in vogue for infants until the seventeenth century when physician and philosopher John Locke and others advocated a more natural and unrestricted childhood.[4]

FROM MYTH TO RELIGION

Sun worship was the foundation for a wide variety of world religions, including Zoroastrianism, Mithraism, Hinduism, Buddhism, Druidism, and European paganism. The Aztecs of Mexico, the Incas of Peru, and many Native American religions also sprang from sun deification. Christianity, too, maintains vestiges of sun worship, largely because at the time it developed, sun-based religions were also soaring in popularity in the Western world.[5]

Cultural appropriation helped smooth the slide from solar worship to Christianity. Beginning in the fourth century, the Christian church moved the celebration of Jesus' birth from January 6 to December 25—a direct challenge to the pagan sun god's popularity. Sunday, the weekly day to celebrate Christian religious worship, was another religious day borrowed from the Mithraists.[6] The winter solstice was called the "Yule" in several languages, which meant "sun." People in as far-flung places as China, Egypt, and Greenland celebrated winter solstice, marked with bonfires, Yule logs, sacrifices, and merry-making. The lighting of a Christmas tree (now strung with electric lights) harks back to pagan solar ceremonies of lit torches, candles, and bonfires, used in midwinter to lure the sun back to life.

SYMBOLISM

The influence of sun-themed symbolism appeared early in human history and persisted, even when submerged beneath the ideology of other religions. Symbols depicting the sun are found in petroglyphs of nearly all societies. The invention of the spoked wheel in 3500 BCE was possibly influenced by the use of circle and spoke images of the sun, which showed up in Neolithic and Early Bronze Age sites.[7] The swastika, a common solar symbol in India and Western Europe, probably originated in symbols of the sun as a wheel. It featured right-handed spokes to symbolically follow the sun's path as it rolled from east to west. The symbol of the cross, too, was initially a solar religious symbol before Christians adopted it. Initially appearing as a combination of a circle and cross, it represented the sun and its extending rays. Similar symbols appear in artifacts found in Asia and the Americas, as well as the Egyptian ankh. Even the shining halo around heads of saints in European paintings represents a solar symbol borrowed from earlier cultures.[8]

The round countenance of the sun itself continues to appear as it once did on petroglyphs. In the 1970s, the ubiquitous "happy face" symbol appeared everywhere and is still present in children's lives, where it's conveyed by authority figures as a mark of approval for behavior or schoolwork well done. Ironically, the sun's symbolism has been co-opted more recently by the largest retailer in the world: WalMart's bright yellow happy face symbol scattered throughout the store assures shoppers they are getting a great buy.

For many of us today, however, the sun holds little meaning in our lives except to brighten our spirits. Technology using solar-powered energy is commonplace in hand-calculators and nightlights; but our focus is elsewhere. We have barely tapped the technological potential of the sun. Creature comforts and responsibilities indoors have lulled us away from sunlight, until we seldom bask in it, preferring our own humanmade controlled environment. Artificial suntan lotions and blonde-streaked hair coloring make the sunless life even easier, so we don't realize that going without UV rays might have an effect on our bodies.

Rather than appreciating the sun and using it to our advantage, we worry about overexposure, skin cancer, and aging. The planet's disappearing protective ozone layer reminds us how vulnerable we are to the power of the sun's ultraviolet radiation, while new health concerns remind us how dependent we are upon that very light.

Chapter Two

A HISTORY OF SUNLIGHT AS THERAPY

Soaking up sunlight is a universal tonic; we're attracted to it and naturally feel better after even a brief exposure. Animals spend hours basking in sun, particularly as they age. Sunlight therapy probably began in the Paleolithic Era, as people basked outside caves to soak up the strengthening rays. The ancient Greeks linked sunlight and healing, best embodied by Aesculapius, the Greek god of medicine, who was also the god of sun and music. While the sun was recognized as a source of heat, it was also a curative. They used the therapeutic power of the sun, notably it's warmth, to treat a variety of diseases, including epilepsy, paralysis, hemorrhage, asthma, jaundice, and obesity. Bathing in springs or seawater was often combined with sunbathing by Greek physicians who sought to bring the body into balance with nature. According to the Greek physician Herodotus, "the sun is especially necessary for people who need restoration and the increase of their muscles." He prescribed guidelines for sunbathing: "one must be careful of the rays which first pass the clouds, and avoid the rays which collect in places protected from the wind." Additionally, "one must take the precaution that in winter, spring and autumn, the sun strike the patients direct; in summer this method must be avoided with weak people; the head must be covered during the treatment."[1] Arab physicians at the time also advised patients to take up sunbathing for asthma, sciatica, and swellings. Sprinkling sand on the skin while sunbathing near the sea was done to make it more comfortable and effective—perhaps it acted as a sunscreen of sorts against burning.

Medical treatment was influenced by politics and religion, and as Christianity grew in popularity, the solar cults and their medicinal use of sunlight eventually faded in the face of medical practices based on prayer and faith. Sunlight therapy disappeared and did not appear again until the nineteenth century. Instead, religious rituals, amulets, and practices like bloodletting and surgical amputation became mainstays of medical treatment, offered by a variety of practitioners sanctioned by the church.

Centuries later, various attempts to resurrect sunlight as a therapeutic or preventive healthcare practice renewed interest in what was viewed as an alternative to traditional medicine. Attempts to revive sunlight therapy in the 1700s were ridiculed; one English physician, Dr. John Lettsome, opened a sun therapy clinic for tuberculosis sufferers but was ridiculed by his colleagues who relied on accepted medical treatments such as phlebotomy and purgatives. He was the butt of the following poem:

> When patients come to I
> I physics, bleeds and sweats 'em
> And if they choose to die
> What's that to I? I Lettsum.[2]

In the 1850s, Jakob Lorber, an Austrian music teacher, garnered a popular following in Germany for his proselytizing about the therapeutic value of sunlight, termed *heliotherapy*. Lorber, acting as a folk practitioner, extolled the healing power of sunlight, advocating sunbathing and drinking water that had been exposed to the rays of the sun. He also created "sun pellets" by exposing milk-based sugar pellets to sunlight, which were proffered as a remedy for many ills.[3] Lacking professional or religious affiliation, however, Lorber's work remained in the realm of folk medicine.[4]

In the nineteenth century, the invention of the microscope allowed people to view live bacteria—the tiny "animalcules" long suspected to exist.[5] Not only could scientists examine these extremely small forms, they could also study the organism's behavior and how they multiplied. The microscope facilitated viewing of sunlight's physical effect on microorganisms. Direct sunlight inhibited the growth of microorganisms in test tubes, and after several hours of exposure, the bacteria disappeared completely. There was no question that light destroyed the bacteria, but how it managed to do so remained a mystery. No one knew whether it was due to the heat or light from ultraviolet radiation. By the 1880s, sunlight's sterilizing effect on water was well known and in the battle against the *bacillus* known as anthrax, scientists recommended cleansing pastures of the spores by cutting down bushes that shaded the grass from sunlight.

Sunlight's use as a therapeutic agent was strengthened by efforts led by German scientist Robert Koch to destroy the deadly bacteria that caused tuberculosis. Although sun therapy had been practiced for centuries, laboratory science began proving its effectiveness. And sunlight treatment seemed to succeed where everything else failed. Tuberculosis—impossible to treat with any existing medical tool—responded to sunlight exposure in the test tube. Laboratory science validated the sun's importance to health and opened it up as a respectable field for scientific research.

A flurry of work followed, using sunlight to eliminate bacteria in water and dozens of other substances. By the mid-1890s, investigations of human urine showed that the bacteria were destroyed by a chemical, not a heat process, as UV light changed urine into hydrogen peroxide. That discovery was followed by work separating the ultraviolet light spectrum by wavelength, from longest to shortest: UV-A, UV-B, and UV-C. Sunlight travels through space in waves of different lengths and UV rays have wavelengths shorter than visible rays. Experiments showed that UV-B rays were more potent against bacteria than UV-A rays, with UV-C rays the strongest of all.[6]

Sunlight can directly affect the growth of some life-forms. Most fascinating, and still under investigation today, was the finding that all cells emit a weak electromagnetic radiation, in a sense communicating with each other. In 1923 scientists discovered that when a protozoan *Paramecium* divides, it emits weak UV rays that stimulate cell division in other *Paramecia*. Exposing *Paramecia* to a small dose of UV radiation from an artificial light stimulated and increased their cell division. Why many types of plant and animal cells (including mammals) emit low-intensity electromagnetic radiation (both visible and UV types) is still not known.[7]

NIELS FINSEN: A NOBEL PRIZE FOR SUNBATHING

In the late nineteenth century, Danish scientist Niels Finsen made the connection between natural sunlight and artificial ultraviolet radiation, thereby proving the value of both as successful medical treatments. He was the first to separate the effect of light from the heat of the sun's rays, identifying the chemical reaction light rays produce in living things as "chemical rays." Finsen came from the northernmost latitudes, the Faroe Islands of the northern Atlantic, and went to medical school in Iceland and Denmark. Never energetic as a child, his health began to fail while he was teaching anatomy at the University of

Copenhagen. He suffered from Pick's disease, a thickening of the connective tissue of membranes in the liver, heart, and spleen. His organs impaired, he developed heart trouble and was eventually confined to a wheelchair. In spite of his handicaps, he pushed himself to learn all he could about the body and its relationship to sunlight, pioneering the use of artificial light as medicine.

Finsen's first work with sunlight was simple: he exposed his forearm to direct summer sun for three hours. The skin blistered with sunburn the next day, except for a strip of skin he had painted with India ink. When the burn faded to a light brown tan, he exposed the arm again, and saw that only the white strip, previously covered by ink, burned this time. He figured something in tanned skin protected it from the sun's rays. He realized sunlight wasn't always harmful, as medical books of the 1890s sometimes claimed; it only harmed skin that wasn't tanned.[8]

He studied the body's reaction to sunlight and ultraviolet radiation from an artificial light source, coming up with a theory that treating smallpox patients with ultraviolet light might prevent pain and scarring common with the disease. He identified the rays from red light as most supportive to the condition, so he used red filters to eliminate the rest of the light spectrum from the treatment process. A few physicians tried the red light treatment on smallpox patients with remarkable results: swelling, fever, and scarring—common with smallpox—didn't occur. More work with smallpox patients showed that they reacted very badly if exposed to ordinary sunlight—they had to be kept in total darkness except for light filtered through a red lens. Many hospitals adopted Finsen's idea, creating "red rooms" where smallpox patients could recover more comfortably. Finsen proved what had been practiced in folk medicine for centuries across Asia and Europe, where the "red treatment" for smallpox patients, a regimen of red drinks and red-dyed clothing, blankets, and curtains, had been adopted as smallpox therapy for generations, but no one knew why it seemed to work. Now, in the age of scientific technology, Finsen had separated the light spectrum with a colored filter and applied it to medicine.[9]

He continued experimenting, next with salamanders in pans of cold water. He reflected sunlight onto their bodies with a mirror that set them swimming when the rays touched them. Then he tried reflecting sunlight through a colored glass filter onto frog embryos in eggs to see how sections of the light spectrum might affect them. Filtering light through blue-green glass made the embryos move around excitedly; changing to red glass, they barely reacted. When a pile of earthworms kept as food for the salamanders appeared dead, he impulsively exposed them to sunlight and almost immediately a few began stretching and squirming, causing him to write, "one can say these chemical rays are life-awakening, energy-stirring . . . a natural force too little noticed in medicine."[10]

Finsen, working without funds or a real laboratory and with only the tools of a schoolboy, had one insurmountable drawback: Denmark's long winters. He began working with an engineer at the local electrical lighting station, trying to find a mechanically generated form of light that could duplicate the rays of the sun so he could work year-round. Carbon arc lights were in common use as street lights because they put out bright, strong light—too intense for home lighting. Arc lights had about two hundred times the illumination power as a filament lightbulb. They consisted of two carbon rods that created a brilliant spark when electric current charged between the two rods. Arc lights were commonly used for outdoor or theater stage lighting, but their brilliance made them ill-suited for homes. By the 1890s, Edison's incandescent lightbulb illuminated homes but arc lights were still in use outdoors. Finsen asked Winfeld Hansen, an engineer at the city light works, to make an arc light strong enough to create a burn, like a sunburn on the body.

Finsen began searching for skin ailments that might respond to light therapy, finding that *lupus vulgaris*, a form of tuberculosis that resulted in small growths on the skin, responded well. In the days before sulfa drugs and antibiotics, the disease disfigured people so badly that surgery was the only solution, but it often left sufferers disfigured or infected. Hansen recruited a friend and fellow engineer named Mr. Mogensen, who suffered from skin tuberculosis for eight years. For two hours every day, from November to March 1896, Finsen treated Mogensen in the city light plant, next to the humming dynamo powering the strong arc light. Using a blue lens, Finsen directed the arc light onto Mogensen's ulcerated face. Results appeared after a month and eventually Mogensen was cured of a disease that had been incurable by every other medical means.[11]

Although successful, Finsen didn't know why it worked. He had applied ultraviolet lamp rays to the patches of patients' infected skin and successfully destroyed the disease-causing agent. At least he thought that's what happened. Rather than sterilize the skin by killing the microbes (as he believed), later experiments by others found that the light treatment bolstered the body's immune system, causing it to heal itself.[12]

But smallpox and skin diseases were only "side-issues" according to Finsen, who lamented that they drew him away from his main focus: proving the beneficial effects of sunbathing. Recognizing that his own health was precarious and that he felt he might not live long enough to spend years in laboratory research, he decided to do clinical experiments using patients of his own. Finsen opened a light therapy clinic in Denmark where patients were treated with natural sunlight outdoors when possible by using large magnifying lenses to capture and focus the ultraviolet rays onto the patient's body. In winter, or when sunlight was unavailable, patients were exposed to specially designed electric lamps, called "Finsen lamps." Using quartz lenses rather than ordinary glass, he concentrated the rays, killing microbes in three seconds. To prevent burning his subjects' skin he filtered the rays through glass tubes full of moving water. During exposure to the "machine-sun," Finsen made patients don lampshade-like headgear to protect their eyes.[13]

His work with artificial light was remarkably successful and captured the interest of scientists and physicians, garnering Finsen the Nobel Prize for Medicine in 1903. With that recognition, sunlight therapy quickly became an acceptable treatment for tuberculosis as well as open wounds. Unable to attend the Nobel awards ceremony to receive his prize, Finsen sent a written speech, explaining what drove him to investigate sunlight. "My disease has played a very great role for my whole development," he wrote. "The disease was responsible for my starting investigations on light." As a youth, he suffered from anemia and lethargy, and while living in a north-facing house, wondered if he would feel better if he received more sun. "I therefore spent as much time as possible in its rays," he explained. He studied everything he could find about the body's reaction to sunlight, but there was so little knowledge available, he found himself venturing onto the new scientific frontier on his own.[14]

He died in September 1904, as summer ended. He left a substantial part of his Nobel Prize award winnings to establish the Finsen Institute in Copenhagen, charged to further the study of light therapy.[15]

Copenhagen was not a very likely location for maximizing therapeutic sunlight, even with the magnifying lenses Finsen fashioned. Switzerland, with higher elevations, lower latitude, and less cloud cover, was a more ideal setting. Auguste Rollier, a Swiss physician, started solar therapy at a sanitarium for sun treatment at Leysen, in the Swiss Alps the year Finsen received his Nobel Prize. Rollier, trained as a surgeon, grew frustrated with orthodox medicine's inability to cure tuberculosis of the skin and joints. Amputating the infected area—the only treatment at the time—left patients without arms and legs; many ultimately choosing suicide to end their misery. In 1903, based on his own empirical observations of sunlight, and empowered by Finsen's Nobel Prize for light medicine, Rollier began sunbath therapy at his own mountain clinic. He treated patients with daily sunbaths, beginning with only twenty minutes of morning sunlight on the patient's feet, the rest of the body covered with a sheet. Sessions gradually progressed to longer exposures up to several hours. The skin progressively tanned and skin sores disappeared.[16]

Rollier went a step farther than Finsen: he not only used sunlight as a curative, he promoted it as a preventive. Calling cities "the suburbs of hell," he treated children who were considered susceptible to tuberculosis because of their generally weakened systems due to urban living. Protective parents enrolled their children at Rollier's boarding school to boost their resistance to illness. The students studied in the open air for two hours a day, wearing only a cotton loincloth, linen hat, and shoes. Rollier's sunlight therapy was so effective he eventually had 3,500 people under his general supervision.[17]

His success was shunned by orthodox medicine, despite the sophisticated new technology in the form of x-rays that helped prove his treatments worked. X-rays clearly showed changes inside the visible body as bones and joints healed and were rebuilt after sun exposure, supporting the value of light therapy.[18]

Light therapy, whether natural or mechanical, was slowly finding its place in medicine. By the late 1920s, physicians in New York and Boston took recovered scarlet fever patients (a highly contagious disease caused by *Streptococcus* bacteria) to Puerto Rico for natural sunlight exposure in winter. Rheumatism, the chronic and debilitating stiffness and swelling of muscles and joints as a result of illnesses such as strep throat infections, was rampant in northern regions, yet unheard of in the sunny south or Puerto Rico.[19] Sunny southern climates in California and New Mexico became popular health meccas.

ILLUMINATION REVOLUTION

Sunlight therapy became popular at a time when most homes had switched to electrical lighting, which extended the hours of work and activity well into the darkness of night. Electrical lighting was a boon in many ways, but people also recognized that it was a powerful force that affected human physiology. Understanding electrical lighting's effect on the body required knowledge about physics and biology that no one had encountered before. Faced with a new technology, public health professionals found themselves challenged to assess the health effects of electrically produced ultraviolet light on the body. If light therapy was so powerful, could the increasingly popular exposure to electric lights in the home cause harm?

Ideas about illumination levels, glare, ultraviolet penetration of the body, and overuse of bright light sources were studied to determine potential effects on the body. In 1924, Janet Clark, a physiological hygiene professor at Johns Hopkins University, examined how levels of illumination affected vision. Myopia—nearsightedness—was linked to using the eyes on close tasks in poor lighting. Although illiterate workers in dimly lit factories suffered from myopia, people generally attributed myopia to literacy, and believed it to be a disease that didn't affect the working classes because they rarely read books. Several researchers linked myopia to indoor professions, pointing out that those who didn't have vision problems usually worked outdoors.[20] Myopia and eyeglasses became commonly accepted as the mark of a studious, educated person.

With brightly lit interiors available at an affordable cost, work could move indoors, windows could be eliminated to save expenses, and workers could continue their tasks well past dusk. As part of the Industrial Revolution, the "Illumination Revolution" changed how, when, and where people worked. In one fell swoop, lighting interior spaces changed urban life immeasurably.

SUN MEDICINE

Ironically, in the 1920s, just as most people were moving indoors for much of the day thanks to interior lighting, sunlight therapy was becoming widely accepted and promised a new frontier in healthcare. "The advent of the sun in scientific medicine is no less glorious than that of the microscope, antisepsis, and anesthesia," one scientific journal enthused. "Its reintroduction into modern therapy is a decided contribution and constitutes a whole new chapter in the history of medical progress."[21] Indeed, it looked extremely promising. As a public health tool against disease and decline, sunlight therapy offered something that was inexpensive, easy to practice, and provided benefits for citizens of all ages. But as simple as it seemed, delivering sunlight to those who needed it most was no easy matter. Wealthy clients could patronize mountaintop clinics and seaside spas; they had the time and money to do so. For working people—many of them children in the days before child labor laws—getting time off work during the day and cash to pay for treatments made sunlight therapy next to impossible. Public health activists provided weekend and summer outings for city dwellers, particularly children, so they could soak up sunshine and fresh air in the country, but it was merely a bandage on a suffering corpse. Poor diets, lack of outdoor recreation facilities, little time, and no money all prevented working-class people from getting the sunshine they needed.

Even for urban children not laboring in factories, there was little that medical science could do to provide sunlight for the children who needed it most. Polluted skies, dark tenements, inadequate amounts of time for playing outdoors, and nonexistent playgrounds made it impossible for many children to overcome their sunlight deficiency. Cod liver oil, which I'll discuss in more detail in chapter 3, provided an inexpensive alternative that worked very well and was widely advertised as a preventive for rickets and general poor health.

MACHINE MEDICINE

But medicine had become a professional field and technology promised to move beyond fish oil tonics for the poor. The era was one of mechanization, machinery, and electricity. Finsen's pioneering use of ultraviolet light and his "sun machine" laid the foundation for a combination of inventions that allowed ultraviolet radiation from artificial lamps to be used as an alternative to natural ultraviolet radiation. Rays from mercury quartz lamps emitted a light wavelength similar to the sun's natural wavelength at the short end of the spectrum. The light itself was too brilliant and powerful for residential lighting but worked well in therapeutic rooms when attendants (and patients) donned protective goggles. Finsen's artificial sunlamps were the initial development in what might be called "machine medicine," which would dominate medical treatments a century later.

Because the reaction to light therapy occurred inside the body and hidden from view, x-rays were invaluable to show before-and-after images of patient's bones. The visible changes in bone ridges could clearly be seen within three weeks of starting light treatment. Ridges along wrists and ankles, common in cases of sunlight deficiency rickets, disappeared after ultraviolet light exposure.[22] Examination of blood samples provided uncontestable proof that sunlight brought about metabolic changes in the human body because lab tests showed clearly that after exposure to mercury quartz lights, blood levels of calcium doubled. Clearly documented changes in the body following light therapy solidified it as an accepted therapeutic. More important at the time, medicine had few other effective treatments to offer for any ailments; sulfa drugs and antibiotics had not yet been discovered.

UV RAYS

Before 1920, research moved ahead due to both serendipity and technology. Separating "heat" rays from "chemical" rays laid the foundation for understanding how sunlight penetrated the body's tissues, creating redness without heat. Early on, the sun's light spectrum was divided into chemical and heat rays, but by the twentieth century, the invisible and violet-blue rays were termed "ultraviolet," while the heat rays were named "infrared radiation." Chemical rays were known to stimulate chemical reactions, for example, their ability to stimulate the conversion of hydrogen and chlorine gases into hydrochloric acid. In the 1880s, recognition that light travels in waves led to a means of measuring smaller microwaves, providing evidence that radiation existed beyond the visible spectrum.

Back in the 1890s, Finsen's work on smallpox had puzzled scientists because red light therapy seemed to help patients by preventing some light rays from reaching the patient. In fact, sunlight was detrimental to smallpox patients. Yet these chemical rays had the opposite effect on tuberculosis of the skin. At the time, no one understood that there were varied portions of the spectrum, or that different parts had different effects on biological processes. After 1909, work by physicists and chemists got a boost from atmospheric scientists who determined the earth's atmosphere reduced UV radiation from the sun by about 40 percent, due to an oxygen layer in the upper atmosphere. Recognition that an ozone filter in the earth's upper atmosphere absorbs most of the sun's UV radiation led to an understanding of the way solar radiation intensity varies throughout the day and with the seasons.[23] By 1920, an understanding of UV radiation and its relationship with sunlight was well established. The commercial and industrial application of UV radiation through means of artificial light sources, along with ways of measuring UV rays, opened the field to scientific medicine.

In the first years of the twentieth century, work from a variety of fields came together and created a better understanding of UV light, yet there was a dark side that was poorly understood. It had long been believed that the warmth from sunlight was the cause of growth and healing in the body. Sunburn and blindness from sungazing were attributed to the heat of the sun. It wasn't until scientists began experimenting with arc lamps and artificial UV light therapy that evidence of harm appeared. Skin burns and eye problems were clearly induced by the chemical rays emitted from artificial light sources because they didn't emit heat. Filtering the light through glass or water (Finsen had tried that) caused less reaction, indicating that it was the rays, not the heat, that served as the active component. In 1896, the first studies of skin cancer in sailors revealed a link between outdoor occupations and skin cancer. The high incidence of cataracts among glass blowers, who were exposed to arc lamps, signaled eye problems due to overexposure to UV rays.[24]

While UV light, whether from sun or artificial lamps, clearly had negative qualities, a consensus developed that sunlight held great value for health. Sunbathing was viewed as a valuable therapeutic practice because it widened or dilated the body's capillaries, increased circulation, and acted as a tonic, restoring muscle tone and resistance to disease. Specific treatment for colitis, rheumatoid arthritis, eczema, lupus, asthma, and even burns was too beneficial to ignore.[25] X-rays and the deleterious effects of the concentrated exposure to such extremely short wavelengths eventually proved how harmful various aspects of radiation treatment could be, but there was little connection between x-rays and basking in natural sunlight.

Both scientific and anecdotal evidence in humans continued to accumulate, adding to a growing body of evidence supporting a therapeutic role for sunlight. Among those who studied disease patterns and the deaths related to them, data charts put together in the late 1920s showed that mortality rates soared during the winter months when little sunlight was available, while these rates dropped to low numbers during the summer. Such broad evidence bolstered the idea that sunlight was another weapon against death and disease.[26] Sunlit rooms, open windows, and taking babies outdoors for daily walks in strollers became hallmarks of effective public health measures. Using sunlight as a tool, one could eliminate bacteria, strengthen the body against disease, and invigorate the mind.

SUNLIGHT AND THE MIND

While direct exposure to light yielded physical results, the effect of general daylight on mental and emotional health hinted that light exposure affected mental ability and mood. Many believed that not only the body, but the mind, too, suffered from the effects of scant sunlight. Mental tests on English school children after outdoor classroom sessions taught in full sunlight showed marked improvement in the test scores of those exposed to sunlight, compared to indoor sessions.[27] The students were more alert and had better coordination of thought and action. In another comparison made on children with pulmonary tuberculosis (the *bacillus* is present in the lungs and lymph nodes), those treated with sunlamps were a year ahead in school achievement when compared to untreated children. The British studies showed the untreated children to be lethargic, unfocused, and inattentive when starting the program, and after sunlight therapy they gained in attention, self-confidence, and enthusiasm for learning.[28] Sunlight's effect on emotional well-being was also recognized, and it was considered a helpful tonic for gloom and depression. It would be decades before circadian rhythms emerged as explanation.

"Sunshine starvation" was evident in modern life, and people and their physicians adopted a variety of ways to remedy the deficiency. During the early decades of the twentieth century, sunlight became a Progressive era mantra: visiting the seaside, walking in the park, or simply opening a window was a conscious act of self-improvement, encouraged by medical and public health professionals. Wealthy homeowners installed glass conservatories in their mansions, and hospitals and sanitariums added sun porches. Enthusiasm for basking in natural sunlight led manufacturers to create a type of window glass that allowed ultraviolet rays to pass through. One hotel in Chicago put the new glass in its guest rooms, and many believed that ordinary window glass would eventually be replaced everywhere by the healthier glass, which didn't screen out ultraviolet rays.[29]

Mindful that modernity limited sunlight exposure, every opportunity to gain sunlight was extolled as a virtue. One could never be too complacent about the advantages of sunlight as well as one's responsibility to seek it out. Even the very popular automobile was quickly identified as a disadvantage to the healthy lifestyle: "the individual who thinks that he is out in the open in his closed automobile fails to realize that it is his car and not he that is getting a sun-bath and the beneficent ultraviolet rays," one magazine noted.[30]

NEW SCIENTIFIC APPROACH

The public accepted its need for sunlight easily. Niels Finsen, his mechanical lighting, and the prestige of his Nobel Prize were pivotal in establishing sunlight as a scientific, rather than a folk-based cure. It was a fact that his protocol was grounded in science and the latest technologies helped prove its value: the microscope, x-rays, chemical assays, electric lights, and statistics all situated sunlight-based therapies into the new scientific paradigm.

To ameliorate winter's darkness, the medical community recognized both artificial light rays and cod liver oil as alternatives to sunlight for children. In 1927, the chairman of the Section on Diseases of Children of the American Medical Association (AMA) said, "Cod liver oil, it seems to me, is our civilization's excellent, economical, and practical substitute—at least during the colder and darker half of the year—for exposure to sunlight. . . . In order to prevent rickets, the administration of cod liver oil or the exposure of the child to the actinic [active radiation] rays should begin early—in our opinion not later than the beginning of the second week of life."[31] For decades, doctors prescribed cod liver oil and many even bottled and sold their own brand to patients.

In the 1920s, physicians embraced artificial light therapy because it was a tool they could offer clients in their own clinics and offices. Light therapy equipment was not costly but did take a skilled practitioner to operate in a manner that prevented burns. It also raised the physician's professional stature in the community and gave patients something that resulted in few ill effects and no obvious dangers.

SUNLIGHT AS PUBLIC HEALTH TOOL

As microscopic medicine began in the nineteenth century, scientists were quick to realize the damaging effects of sunlight and UV rays on single-celled organisms such as bacteria. Even before the sunlight research on animals and humans began, scientists could see that microorganisms either thrived in light or were harmed by it. In the 1880s, direct sunlight was applied to anthrax spores, typhus bacteria, and tetanus—effectively killing them all. In 1888, a French scientist used sunlight to sterilize water, suggesting cities adopt ultraviolet light to purify drinking water. One researcher discovered sunlight's bactericidal quality extended beneath the surface of water, to a depth of half a meter. In 1943, *E. coli*, a bacterium naturally resident in the human gut but also a dangerous toxin in food products, was killed with intense ultraviolet light in experiments laying the groundwork for irradiation as a food sanitizer.[32]

In the years between the rise of bacteriology in the late nineteenth century and the development of sulfa drugs and antibiotics in the mid-twentieth century, awareness of sunlight's cleansing properties was quickly accepted by public health advocates who pushed for the use of sunlight as a tool to clean up dirty tenements. The Progressive era saw many efforts to improve sanitation, city neighborhoods, and public health standards, and professionals wanted to move beyond soap and water as weapons in the fight against germs. The sun's ultraviolet radiation proved an excellent agent. In the 1920s, new work on sunlight therapy led many to view it as an effective agent against nearly all diseases. Some viewed malaria, for example, as caused by the stimulation of sunlight radiation because the disease was more common in spring and summer—the sunny season. Others thought pellagra, a deficiency disease related to lack of niacin, might be caused by the effects of sunlight on the bodies of people who had consumed an unknown toxin in corn. It took time and work to find the answers to malaria and pellagra, and in neither case was sunlight involved. Tuberculosis, however, a common problem in that era, responded so well to sunlight exposure that UV light treatments became standard therapy for the disease.

QUESTIONS REMAINED

Light therapy was powerful and puzzling. It clearly changed bodies, tissues, and cells—that was evident in laboratory work. But how it did so, and most important, how light rays appeared to alter metabolic processes deep within the body—without burning the surface tissues—remained a mystery. Patients responded to ultraviolet light, but how the body processed the light falling on the skin's surface was unknown. How ultraviolet light could be therapeutic, yet not appear to penetrate the skin, was the mystery.

Chapter Three

DOGS IN THE DARK
AND THE DISCOVERY OF VITAMIN D

In the 1930s, Weston A. Price, a dentist from Cleveland, visited Auguste Rollier's alpine sun clinic while traveling to assess health and diet in various settings around the world. Long forgotten—even ignored—Price's observations about health and diet today inspire thousands of devotees seeking improved health by eating traditional rather than processed foods. Price's work has been revived today through the efforts of the Price-Pottenger Foundation and the Weston A. Price Foundation, groups advocating a return to a diet of whole foods, foods that have been unprocessed such as fruits, vegetables, and fresh meats.

Also during the 1930s, Price tried to unravel the reason for the growing amount of tooth decay in industrial societies. A dentist-cum-anthropologist, he visited isolated sites around the world, looking for indigenous people still eating their traditional diets. He also chronicled physical changes in groups that had switched from traditional indigenous diets to processed foods, taking voluminous photographs to support his findings. He found that dental decay was caused primarily by nutritional deficiencies, the same deficiencies that create general poor health.

Traditional diets conferred immunity to dental decay and disease, yet those diets varied greatly, depending on geography and environment. The only commonalities he found among diets of healthy groups were the use of animal products and salt. He analyzed the foods and found that traditional peoples were eating four times the amount of vitamins and minerals as Americans at the time. Price focused on fat-soluble vitamins, recognizing they were a key component of healthy diets. He found them most abundant in butterfat, fish oils, organic meats, fish, eggs, and animal tallow (lard).

Price made an interesting observation about the patients at Rollier's alpine clinic: none of the patients came from the isolated Alpine valleys where people were still eating traditional high-calcium diets. Those mountain dwellers relied on rye bread and cheese, not the processed foods that had become popular in the low-lying towns, and consequently they had superior teeth and stature. Price attributed their good health to their traditional dairy-based high-calcium diet, along with plenty of sunlight and the higher amount of UV rays at higher elevations.

In communities where children ate white bread and drank milk from cows kept indoors in barns, Price found a quarter of the children's teeth had decayed to the gum line. He wrote that to alleviate the tooth decay problem, schoolchildren should be allowed more opportunity to get sunlight, dress in sun suits, and play outdoors before lunch each day.[1] Physicians and dentists in Switzerland told Price that tuberculosis and dental caries were usually linked, in turn, supporting his research that dietary calcium was integral to health.[2]

Price believed that sunlight and nutrition were being accepted too simplistically. There was much to explore, he argued, pointing out that butter from cows grazed on green grass in spring contained mysterious health-giving components, far beyond what had been recognized. He referred to the complex as "activator X," and chronicled examples of its curative powers on many malnourished American children he treated during the Great Depression.[3]

BEGINNINGS OF NUTRITIONAL SCIENCE

Price's observations remain provocative and valuable, yet to fully appreciate his findings, we must look at the underpinnings of modern nutritional science and its emergence in the first decades of the twentieth century. Throughout history, people always connected food to health but believed it was simply a matter of getting enough to eat. Quantity rather than quality was the accepted standard, justifiably so because food was often scarce. The common assumption was that those who could afford to eat the most food ate better. But as the nineteenth century passed into the twentieth, industrialization and railroad transportation made commercially processed food more available, until finally urban factory workers purchased everything they ate. No longer did most people rely on the family milk cow or the vegetable garden. Canned and salted foods, cereals, and sugars were affordable, and when bolstered by advertising in the growing number of popular magazines, they became attractive alternatives to labor-intensive farming and food preparation practices. Colorful labels on cans of vegetables sported glorious images of an agrarian Eden, and ads reassured consumers that processed foods were as good as or even superior to fresh ones. Consumers worried more about getting cheated by adulterated products than about what nutrients they might not be getting. People expected to get their money's worth in the marketplace and that meant taste and purity—nutritive value was still a foggy concept. While staple foods were more available and cheaper, the quality of most people's diets actually declined.

The beginning of a nutrition-based approach to diet came from the age of exploration, when sailors confined to meager diets aboard ship developed a host of nutrient-deficient conditions. In 1536, French sea explorer Jacques Cartier attempted to find a Northwest Passage when 110 members of his crew developed scurvy (i.e., swollen gums, loose teeth, and bleeding under the skin), a common and dangerous problem in the age of sailing ships. Native Americans living in what is now Canada introduced him to a tea made of bark and needles from the White Pine tree—rich in ascorbic acid (vitamin C)—and the crew recovered. Cartier didn't find a passage and his notes concerning the tonic went unnoticed. In 1753, James Lind, a British naval doctor, rediscovered Cartier's notes and began experimenting with the diet of sailors aboard ship. He discovered that fresh vegetables, cider, and oranges seemed to alleviate scurvy symptoms and kept men alive longer. His efforts were ignored at the time, but eventually the British Navy adopted citrus fruits, giving each sailor a ration of lime juice, earning them the nickname, "limeys." But the solution was purely empirical—no one understood why certain fresh vegetables or fruits cured scurvy, or even what caused it to develop in the first place. In 1840, a physician predicted that scurvy was "due to the lack of an essential element which it is hardly too sanguine to state will be discovered by organic chemistry of the experiments of physiologists in a not too distant future."[4] His prediction was correct, but it took scientists about a hundred years to figure out why.

The weakness, wasting, and nerve damage of beriberi was another chronic complaint that afflicted ship's crews, particularly on Japanese ships. In 1878, the director-general of the Japanese navy suspected it was related to diet, so he added evaporated milk and meat to the sailors' diet of milled rice. When his crew recovered, he attributed it to the protein supplements. In 1896, Christiaan Eijkman, a military doctor, recognized the real problem, lack of vitamin B (thiamin) due to removal of the rice husks during milling. He discovered the difference when he switched the diet of his hospital's chicken flock to milled rice, which caused them to develop symptoms of beriberi. Calling the syndrome "partial hunger," Eijkman's ideas were scorned at first but laid the groundwork for further investigation. Years later, in 1929, Eijkman received the Nobel Prize for his discovery of what became known as vitamins.

LIEBIG'S SIMPLE ELEMENTS A FAILURE

Meanwhile, chemists—particularly German ones—were making great strides in understanding the relationship between food and metabolism, or how the body converts what we eat into energy. Justus von Liebig, the foremost chemist of the age, discovered in the 1890s that foods were made up of four main elements: carbohydrate, protein, fat, and minerals. He believed that the key to a proper diet was simply to combine the elements in appropriate amounts. However intuitive his original hypothesis was, Liebig's quantitative and reductionist approach did not work when applied. The elements alone could not simply be combined to formulate nutritional fare.

J. B. H. Dumas, a French physician, discovered that creating an artificial diet along the lines proposed by Liebig didn't work. In 1871, while Paris was under siege by German soldiers, Dumas saw firsthand how devastating a synthetic diet could be when he tried to create food to feed starving infants in an orphanage. Trying to reconstruct food from other materials, he combined appropriate amounts of emulsified fat in a sweetened solution of water and egg whites, creating what technically was artificial milk. The infants failed to thrive, and the sad situation convinced Dumas there was some other undiscovered substance in milk that was essential to life.

DISCOVERY OF VITAMINS

Casimir Funk, a Polish researcher working in Europe, pulled together the scattered experimental work done with animal diets and theorized that beriberi, scurvy, pellagra, and maybe even rickets were caused by the lack of some "special substances" in foods, which he named *vital amines*, or "vitamines." Funk's paper, published in the *Journal of State Medicine* in 1912 and widely read, caused a sensation. Funk did not come up with the idea in a vacuum; he picked up the thinking of several others who suspected there were unidentified nutrients in foods. Sporadic work on food and diet by several researchers had hinted that something beyond Liebig's four elements was present in foods and essential for a healthful diet, and the time had come to establish a theoretical framework for further investigation. Scurvy, which could be cured with lemons, and beriberi, with whole rice, had been resolved as food-related illnesses that could be treated with diet. While both diseases could clearly be either prevented or cured by consumption of specific foods, there had been no sound theory or proof behind the use of lemons or whole rice. Deficiency in the diet was an entirely new concept. After Funk's paper appeared, several other researchers published work they had done years before, having been reluctant to expose their work in light of strong disapproval from the nutritional science establishment.[5]

"That notion—that disease was due to a *lack*—involved a new paradigm," medical historian Roy Porter explains. The nineteenth century had been the age of the microscope and microbes, as laboratory scientists took the lead in explaining disease. Metabolism was believed to be a chemical process reduced to Liebig's theory, and disease was viewed as a microbe problem. Chemists and physicians thought they had little in common. Each had their own problems to solve, but who would imagine their fields of study might entwine? Indeed, they sometimes were at odds in explaining the causes of diseases.[6]

But Funk and others were part of a worldwide realization that food and disease were linked somehow through metabolism. But there was so little understood about both metabolism and nutrient composition of food that it would take decades to build a solid knowledge of nutrition. And because most deficiency diseases were linked to poverty, there was little incentive to act on the clinical knowledge once it was established.

Without adequate scientific understanding of metabolism, demagogues and snake oil hucksters continued to drive nutrition science, and Americans literally ate it up. The discovery of nutrients in foods launched a variety of dietary regimens, tonics, and supplements. Identifying, isolating, and studying the composition of foods became a new frontier in science and medicine. If one could determine which foods held essential nutrients, people could reshape their diets for maximum health.[7]

NORWAY'S REMEDY

Along with the multitude of proprietary tonics and elixirs, a traditional folk cure came into popular use. Cod liver oil, a Norwegian folk remedy, using smelly oil extracted from the innards of codfish, cured rickets. It was a popular, if nauseating, treatment, but it worked and pushed scientists to ask whether rickets might be a dietary disorder. Cod liver oil wasn't a protein or carbohydrate and the body's response to it was unlike that to any other fat or oil. Other oils, such as butter or olive oil, had no effect on ailments like rickets and gout, while empirical evidence showed cod liver oil cured both. Cod liver oil, doled out to children and adults alike to regain health, was a reminder that chemistry had not answered all the questions about food composition.

In Norwegian fishing villages, cod liver oil's remarkable qualities had been relied on for generations, based on the traditional knowledge that cod liver oil makers were never ill. Used to light lamps all over Europe, for centuries the smelly oil was Norway's most valuable export commodity. The traditional extraction process relied on slow fermentation, but in 1854, a Norwegian pharmacist built special kettles to boil fresh fish livers, speeding up the process. The oil rose to the top of the cauldron where it was skimmed off and bottled. He won awards at trade fairs across Norway and launched a new industry in a country with few commercial options. It came at the right time—commercially prepared medicinal cod liver oil entered the marketplace as Europe and Britain experienced a rise in chronic illness due to the Industrial Revolution.[8]

Cod liver oil was inexpensive, could be easily dosed at home, and cured ailments more often than the medical profession's standard treatments such as bloodletting and mercury potions. Doses of cod liver oil restored health in a variety of situations and continued to remind scientists that there was something else in foods—something vitally important—besides Liebig's four components.

OILS AND FATS

As scientists explored food composition in the laboratory, increasing knowledge only revealed more challenges to identifying and understanding these minute components in foods. Fats were especially confounding. Tests with various cooking oils and animal fats revealed that not all fats were alike. Some fats contained a substance the others lacked—something that was essential to health in laboratory animals. Understood to act as a "fuel" food, researchers realized fats were more complex. Elmer McCollum and Marguerite Davis, working at the University of Wisconsin in 1913, found that laboratory rats on restricted diets developed eye problems, which could then be cured by adding butterfat to their diet. The mysterious essential element was termed "fat-soluble A," a nomenclature that paved the way for a series of nutrients given alphabetic names.[9] Casimir Funk, building upon Eijkman's work identifying the missing component in processed rice that caused beriberi, isolated an essential element in rice husks and yeast, which he called "water-soluble B." A third entity found in certain fruits and vegetables was known to cure scurvy but was different from vitamin A or B; it was named vitamin C, the next letter in the alphabet.

Blindness, beriberi, and scurvy: the new chemistry of vitamins promised to eliminate them all. The next nutrient to be identified would naturally be called "D." Identifying vitamin D was merely the threshold to understanding it, however. Solving the mystery of vitamin D took the fields of chemistry, biology, and physics nearly a century to figure out.

THE ENGLISH DISEASE

In 1911, Britain inaugurated the National Health Insurance Act. Along with contributions to their own immediate healthcare, each person insured under the act contributed one penny annually to fund medical research. When World War I broke out three years later, the nation's health status was crucial to national defense. It was immediately clear that the young working-class men the nation relied upon for military recruits were in poor health. The government created a list of the country's major disabling diseases and invited medical researchers to select which one they wanted to investigate. Tuberculosis, rheumatism, chronic arthritis, rickets, and dental disease topped the list. Rickets, an affliction so common in Britain it had long ago been termed "the English Disease," was particularly important because it affected the working-class youth who would be the nation's military strength.[10]

Prevalent and worrisome, rickets had been the subject of much attention for decades. It was apparent there was a strong geographic or environmental connection. Historically, rickets had been considered a disease that affected children of the wealthy, who spent their time indoors, but with the advent of the Industrial Revolution, the problem seemed to expand to the urban poor.[11] Cases were found more frequently in cities and large towns, particularly where industry was located, and seldom in the rural areas. It was rampant in the industrial towns and coal districts in both England and Scotland. The Scottish Highlands were virtually free of it, however. In London proper, the wealthy neighborhoods were free of it, and the number of cases declined as one moved from the city to the outlying regions.

Rickets appeared to be linked in some way to population density and afflu-ence because residents in small villages or in wealthy city neighborhoods seldom experienced it. Many theorists focused on crowded living conditions as the cause, basically due to factors such as inadequate sanitation and poverty. But a medical consensus didn't emerge. The 1911 edition of *Encyclopaedia Britannica* attributed rickets to a toxin in the digestive tract.[12] Tiny Tim, the crippled boy in *A Christmas Carol* by Charles Dickens, written in 1843, per-sonified the child with rickets. Using a crutch and an iron frame supporting his limbs, helpless Tiny Tim linked rickets to poverty in the public's mind.

But poverty was not the cause, many argued. To make it even more baf-fling, rickets occurred among the poor in Beirut but also among the wealthy in Egypt. It was uncommon among the poor in Latin America, California, and the West Indies. For years, the geographic distribution of rickets continued to stymie the medical community. It was well known that the incidence was higher in temperate latitudes—there were few cases in Greenland or Iceland in the far north, and few in southern latitudes such as southern Spain, Turkey, and Greece. While not as prevalent as in Great Britain, rickets was found in a swath across Germany, England, Holland, Belgium, France, and northern Italy. Cold, wet climates were suspect, as well as the soil in damp regions. In fact, one sci-entist believed it to be a form of malaria.

Rickets was prevalent in the United States, as well, although there it did not garner much attention from the medical community. It was commonly found in Philadelphia and Boston in numbers equivalent to England.[13]

In the 1880s, Theobald Palm, an English physician, embarked on a global epidemiological effort to solve the mystery of rickets and wrote to missionaries around the world for information about rickets in their areas. Palm corre-sponded with missionary physicians in Mongolia and in both urban and rural

China. None reported any cases of rickets. Some attributed its absence to the hard mineral water, which contained calcium. In Tibet, a physician extolled the virtues of the elevation, which at over eleven thousand feet appeared to be responsible for eliminating most diseases entirely. "Were our hills not so difficult of access, we might start a sanatorium for all sorts of complaints of men," he noted.[14] In India, cases of rickets were common among weavers, who spent most of their lives indoors, and in the urban areas of Punjab. But this was an isolated disease population. Nearly everyone else the missionary doctors encountered spent most of their day outdoors: from the poor working or basking in the sun, to the wealthy on patios or open inner courtyards. One writer told Palm that the only people he thought did not go outdoors were the "inmates of the zenana"—referring to the secluded part of the house where females spent their time in Moslem homes—but he lamented that he had no access to the women's quarters to assess their health status.[15]

Another physician, William Huntley, a native of Glasgow, Scotland, working in India, wrote that the operation of osteotomy, which was common in Scotland, was never needed in India. Osteotomy is a surgical procedure to straighten a crooked bone; the bone is sliced in half, then realigned and allowed to heal. A severe treatment for the misshapen bones of rickets, it was commonly performed by Scottish surgeons. Huntley described people in India living in abject poverty and filth, with diets made up largely of barley, who nevertheless did not develop rickets. "What have they then to counterbalance the evil of the filth and dirt surrounding them?" he asked. "The answer I think, is sunlight." He described the lack of ventilation in the foul-smelling huts where he treated patients in India, and explained, "The grand counterbalancing fact which stands out is the sunlight. Natives rich and poor, old and young, spend most of the day in the sunlight and the open air."[16]

Palm's global research refuted some of the long-held theories about rickets in Britain. Some experts blamed the venereal disease syphilis for the debilitating symptoms of rickets, but syphilis was common in Morocco and Japan, where rickets was unknown. Others blamed poverty, yet some of the most destitute children in the tropical world lived free of the disease while it ran rampant in Britain, the world's wealthiest nation at that time.[17] Clearly, whatever caused rickets transcended sanitation measures, and no infectious agent seemed to be involved. Because nutritional research was a new frontier, the question of diet or dietary deficiencies arose, but that, too, seemed to be a dead end. British children, even those in the working class, were considerably better fed than those in the teeming slums of Calcutta—who did not suffer from rickets. It could not be diet alone.

Like Huntley, Palm noted that the one common denominator found in all regions where rickets was nonexistent was abundant sunshine. The problem appeared related to British fog and the perennial pall of coal smoke, made worse by the habit of building three-story buildings that shaded the ground from any sunlight that might appear. Poor children spent their time outdoors in dark alleys or indoors with their mothers doing homebound piecework such as sewing, folding paper flowers, or rolling cigars. Palm urged scientists to study the physiological and therapeutic actions of sunlight, noting that recent findings in organic chemistry revealed the profound effect of sunlight on plant life. Physicians, he declared, should educate the public about the importance of sunlight to health, noting that people seemed to prefer staying inside their dwellings, with the "carpets and curtains," rather than outdoors. Sunlight, he pointed out, "is nature's universal disinfectant, as well as a stimulant and tonic." Palm believed that clearing up the polluted air, expanding the number of open spaces in cities, and creating playgrounds for children of the poor would eliminate rickets.[18]

WORLD WAR I SPURS DISCOVERY OF VITAMIN D

Eventually, war spurred research that led to an understanding of nutrient deficiency. In 1914, as wartime fears prompted attention to medical problems of the general population in England, Edward Mellanby, a professor of pharmacology at the University of Sheffield, and his wife, May, a professor in the Household and Social Science Department of London University, chose to investigate rickets as part of the national health research program. They worked at a laboratory in their country home studying puppies, which were known to sometimes develop rickets. Their approach was to create rickets in dogs using experimental diets of various components. They fed different groups of dogs strictly controlled diets based on combinations of skim milk, oil (butter, lard, olive oil, or cod liver oil), orange juice, yeast, cereal (white flour, rice, oatmeal, corn), and some lean meat. They discovered that the type of fat used in the diet made the difference. Animal fats, such as lard or fish oil, had no detrimental effect on the puppies, but the groups fed vegetable oils developed soft, deformed bones. The Mellanbys suspected that rickets was due to a dietary deficiency of a fat-soluble vitamin, such as vitamin A or something similar to it. Eventually they identified two separate nutrients: an "anti-infective agent" that thwarted infections (vitamin A) and a "calcifying vitamin" that would later be identified as vitamin D.[19]

The Mellanbys found other results at the conclusion of their experiment. A bevy of health conditions emerged that had not been recognized as connected to rickets previously, including: sensitivity to anesthetics, heightened anxiety, and lowered resistance to infection, which are all common to animals deficient in a fat-soluble vitamin.[20]

TOOTH DECAY

May Mellanby noticed something else during the experiments: the puppies that experienced weakened bones also developed badly decayed teeth. She concluded that animal products such as milk, eggs, fish oil, and butter produced animals with well-formed teeth, while more exclusively, cereal diets formed defective teeth. Her findings pointed to the general problem of defective teeth among British citizens, due both to poor diet by the mother while pregnant as well as poor general nutrition.[21]

May Mellanby's article, "The Influence of Diet on Teeth Formation," appeared in the British medical journal the *Lancet* in December 1918. She challenged the dental health community to consider nutrition as a factor in caries development, but her suggestion was not immediately accepted because other theories, based on bacteria and food textures as stimulants to tooth decay, held sway. At the time, the idea that incidence of dental cavities could be measured, or even prevented, was an open question.[22] May Mellanby then looked at "the etiology of hypoplasia"—how teeth develop from inside the body. Instead of hygiene, she proved that diet controls tooth development and some factor in the diet controlled calcification of the teeth. She termed this unknown factor a *vitamine*, using Casimir Funk's term. The factor was vitamin D, in the form of cod liver oil.

May Mellanby explained that "One can now see a rather obscure but still a real picture illustrating the cause of the defective teeth of modern civilization. . . . Our diet, especially that of the poor, is made up of specially prepared cereals, such as wheat, rice, oats, etc. Meat and the animal fats tend to play a smaller part." She noted that the Eskimo in the far north, "where flesh and blubber are the staple articles of diet, have such excellent teeth," while other cultures who subsisted on mostly grains had terrible teeth.

Her work was groundbreaking, but she could not clearly identify what the missing vitamin was. She believed it was vitamin A, which indeed was found in animal fats. Not realizing that there was a specific component in fish oil, she thought "the teeth of the people of this country will tend to become worse unless our diet consists in the future more of whole milk and other foods containing fat-soluble vitamine A and less of bread, rice, potatoes, and etc., which are deficient in this factor." Cod liver oil itself made the experimental results difficult to define because it contained large amounts of both vitamin A and vitamin D. The Mellanbys, on the frontier of fat-soluble vitamin research, found that results between fats varied. For example, butter was a good source of vitamin A, while lard contained little A or vitamin D (called "factor X," at the time). Cod liver oil was the only fat they tested that contained both A and "factor X" in significant amounts.[23]

While the Mellanbys identified cod liver oil as a curative for rickets, they were confused because it seemed to have another component besides the antirickets factor that prevented pneumonia and eye problems in rachitic dogs (afflicted with rickets). In 1922, Elmer McCollum, professor of biochemistry at Johns Hopkins Medical School, led investigations using oxygen bubbled through cod liver oil, identifying two separate components: vitamin A and vitamin D.[24]

Fat, cereal-fed babies were weak physically, causing speculation that a grain-based diet lacked something elemental. Edward Mellanby found that besides promoting weight gain, grains such as wheat flour, oatmeal, rice, and corn appeared to play a role in preventing calcification of bones in experiments feeding controlled diets to dogs. He found oatmeal to be the worst offender, but his findings were rejected at a Glasgow meeting of the British Medical Association. Physicians continued to argue against diet having anything to do with rickets and bristled at the insinuation that Scotland's national food—oatmeal—might be to blame. Overcrowded living conditions, defective hygiene, and lack of exercise were the causes for rickets, his critics insisted. As Mellanby later remarked, the resistance to his ideas was strong. "The new indictment at Glasgow of the Scottish national food, oatmeal, as the king of rickets-producers roused much emotion, among both those participating in the research and the onlookers," he wrote.[25]

Oatmeal had been the staple food in Scotland for as long as anyone could remember, and the Scots were known for their sturdy physical strength and stamina. They took a backseat to no other group as far as health. It seemed too far-fetched to blame the epidemic of rickets rampant in the industrial areas on oatmeal. Mellanby himself realized it hardly made sense, but he explained that it might be because the Scots had changed how they ate—no longer did they consume large quantities of fresh milk with oatmeal. Few city-dwellers even had access to a milk cow or fresh milk. And the demise of fishing villages meant fewer people consumed large quantities of fish. Mellanby tried to explain that it wasn't oatmeal's fault that Scottish children grew up misshapen. There was an underlying lack of something in children's diets, which eating oatmeal simply exacerbated. If Scots continued relying on cereal for the bulk of their diet, they had to find ways to supplement it with whatever nutrient was missing.

Through their restricted diet research, the Mellanbys had identified phytic acid, a naturally occurring phosphorus compound found in cereal grains, legumes, and nuts. Phytates bind with minerals such as iron, calcium, and zinc and interfere with their absorption in the body. Phytates are degraded by yeast and enzymes in bread making and destroyed by baking. Phytates in grains are also destroyed during sprouting, roasting, and fermentation. What the Mellanbys called "the cereal factor" was phytic acid, a component of grain that prevents the utilization of calcium and phosphorus. By 1922, they had also identified the elusive fat-soluble nutrient vitamin D, which not only prevented rickets but counteracted phytic acid's action on calcium and phosphorus in the diet.[26]

THE DARKNESS EFFECT

What the Mellanbys tended to ignore, however, was that the reason they were able to induce rickets in dogs was because they purposely reared them indoors. Lack of sunlight caused rickets; the discovery of cod liver oil as a dietary form of vitamin D was an attempt to provide a naturally occurring form of a substance also created by sunlight.

The Glasgow physicians, who argued against oatmeal as a rickets factor, thought sunlight and fresh air were more important than diet in curing rickets.

In this case, both the Mellanbys and the physicians were right. When sunlight was deficient, rickets developed. It was exacerbated by a grain diet and cured by fat-soluble vitamin D, found in cod liver oil. Healthy outcomes required both sunlight and proper diet.

HELIOPATHY: SUN AND LIGHT CURES

As soon as World War I ended, a British medical group went to Vienna to assist relief efforts among the poor. The prevalence of rickets was high in the devastated postwar economy. Physician Harriette Chick, a member of the British group, began dosing Viennese children suffering from rickets with cod liver oil. Chick confirmed the Mellanbys' work, finding that the only children who recovered from rickets in winter were those given cod liver oil. In summertime, however, when the children could be outdoors, they recovered without the aid of cod liver oil, proving the value of natural sunlight. Dr. Chick conducted several similar experiments, concluding that summer sunlight had a curative effect.[27]

Karl Huldschinsky, a pediatrician in Germany after the war, also took on rickets, which was rampant among German children at the time. He examined youngsters between the ages of three and five years at Berlin's Oscar-Helene Home for Crippled Children. All of his subjects had severely deformed limbs and curved spines, delayed growth, and active rickets. He discovered that one rachitic child recovered after exposure to a quartz mercury vapor lamp treatment and began experimenting on fifty children, using sunbaths and exposure to artificial light. He used the new technology of x-rays to prove that the children's bones healed, but he could do nothing to straighten their misshapen limbs once growth had taken place. Unable to alter the aftereffects of rickets, he decided that prevention was crucial. "It is true that I had healed the bones, but I had not cured the deformities in them," he wrote in 1927. "The conclusion I came to was that it is not much good curing rickets unless one cures the disease before the bones have become deformed; so my first postulate was the paradoxical one that to cure rickets one must prevent rickets occurring."[28]

He gave younger children ultraviolet light treatments as preventive measures, hoping to stave off rickets before the condition advanced. His work added to the knowledge about healthy growth, proving that both cod liver oil (and its mysterious vitamin D component) and sunlight (or ultraviolet lighting) could arrest or prevent rickets.[29]

Huldschinsky understood what the Mellanbys had largely overlooked in their focus on dietary factors in disease prevention: that sunlight was key. Like Palm and others before him who had touted sunlight to prevent rickets, Huldschinsky focused on light, and more significantly, artificial light, in his therapeutic protocol. The application of artificial light, using the new technology of the time, gave Huldschinsky's work immediacy and importance. Rather than pointing to natural sunlight as a solution, which wasn't practical in urban areas covered in the pall of industrial smoke, Huldschinsky's use of artificial ultraviolet lighting stimulated the rest of the scientific community because it used technologies that were so new they were little understood. He built on Finsen's work, linking UV light therapy to disorders inside the body—not just on the skin's surface. His documentation through x-rays showed clear results at bone remineralization after ultraviolet light treatments.

The adoption of both x-rays and quartz mercury lightbulbs was a turning point in controlling the body's exposure to ultraviolet light. Therapeutic artificial light treatment could be supported by clear evidence in x-ray images of the changes in the bones. Huldschinsky's work brought what had been largely a folk cure (sunbathing) into mainstream scientific medicine because its results were measurable and documented visually.

Almost concurrently with Huldschinsky's experiments in Germany, two New York City physicians, Alfred Hess and L. J. Unger, added another dimension to understanding rickets. Their laboratory experiments with rats revealed that minerals were somehow involved because rats that developed rickets on a diet adequate in calcium but lacking in phosphorus recovered when given either phosphorus or sunlight exposure.[30] Given the Viennese and German results, the solution to rickets seemed within grasp, but the implications of Hess and Unger's findings baffled researchers. Their results shed a disturbing new light on sun exposure and rickets. Diet and sunlight apparently offered separate paths to both preventing and curing inadequate bone development. Yet the two were somehow connected. How could such different factors as cod liver oil, sunlight, minerals, and mercury vapor lightbulb rays all have the same effect on the body?

Deciphering how such disparate elements as sunlight and fish oil could have similar effects on metabolism and growth seemed impossible. In 1925, two biophysicists at Harvard explained that "while the clinicians of the past century were experimenting with cod liver oil, the presence or absence of sunlight was affecting their results without their knowledge, and thus causing confusion." The professors, Wallace Craig and Morris Belkin, noted that it took years to recognize that invisible rays from sunlight couldn't pass through window glazing. Patients given sunbaths outdoors improved, while those exposed indoors to sunlight rays filtered through window glass did not, thereby supporting theorists who claimed the health benefits of a "sunbath" came from fresh air—not sunlight. Theobald Palm's work stood alone—and unproven—as the only systematic work supporting sunlight rather than fresh air or other factors.

A CHEAPER ALTERNATIVE: IRRADIATED FOODS

During the post-World War I years, treating babies with sunlight worked well, but clinically it was expensive, difficult to control, and not very scientific. Besides, impoverished urban infants at risk for rickets were not likely to be given daily sunbaths, even if the skies were clear. Crowded apartment buildings towered over the streets and luxuries like city parks—and the time to enjoy them—were scanty. Finding a cheap dietary alternative to natural sunlight would be the most economical alternative. Treating inexpensive foods with sunlight—if it worked—would be a perfect solution.

Experiments performed on laboratory animals, irradiating the animals themselves at first and eventually their foods, provided convincing evidence that ultraviolet radiation was key to curing and preventing rickets. Ultraviolet exposure from a quartz light altered cotton seed and linseed (flax seed) oils, making them just as efficient at curing rickets in rats as doses of cod liver oil.

At the University of Wisconsin–Madison, experiments with rats confirmed that their entire diet could be irradiated successfully for the prevention of rickets-like bone disease. These findings set off a flurry of irradiated food experiments, the most successful of which involved natural oils, such as olive oil, corn oil, lard, and butter. Irradiating mineral oil did not work, and neither did sugar, but cereals, vegetables, and egg yolk could be treated with ultraviolet light to produce the elusive element that bones needed. Milk, the most popular source of calcium, was also irradiated following pasteurization. In the United States, even irradiated and reconstituted dry milk powder proved successful at preventing rickets.

Food irradiation was almost too good to be true: middle-class children thrived on diets of cereal and milk, which had been considered a poor diet before irradiation changed the nutrient content of the milk, turning it into "liquid sunshine." Later the fortification of milk with vitamin D, along with commercial homogenization and pasteurization, bolstered the growing breakfast cereal industry that rose out of John Harvey Kellogg's enterprising efforts at Battle Creek, Michigan, after the turn of the century.[31]

Like today, irradiated food was not accepted without question. In Germany, protests arose after publications warned of damaging health effects to mice and guinea pigs fed irradiated milk. Irradiated milk had a bad taste, too, described as "fishiness or rancidity." In the irradiation process, milk was exposed to light for periods of between five and twenty minutes, often souring it in the process. Oils and grains were exposed for up to thirty minutes. The food, in a thin layer not more than an eighth of an inch thick, was passed slowly beneath a quartz mercury vapor lamp positioned about two feet away. Once properly treated by artificial light, foods retained the nutritional value of the as yet elusive vitamin D permanently, despite long storage periods or high cooking temperatures. Problems arose, however, because there wasn't a standardized method for administering the UV treatment or its results. Food products could attain very high levels of vitamin D—or none at all. Over time, methods were refined and eventually patented.

In 1925, chemist Harry Steenbock, lead researcher at the University of Wisconsin, patented the process of treating food by ultraviolet light and assigned the patent to the Wisconsin Alumni Research Foundation. The nonprofit foundation licensed manufacturers and controlled their production and advertising. The university had earlier set a precedent for public research when it developed the Babcock test, an innovative yet simple test for butterfat content in milk. Both procedures saved consumers money and improved health. By holding the patent for irradiation, the school profited and prevented private interests from monopolizing the process. In 1927, the Quaker Oats Company was first to sign on with the foundation to purchase irradiation rights for its cereals. The Fleischmann Company followed, selling irradiated yeast.

Neither altruism nor regulation prompted food processors to jump on board the fortification bandwagon; rather, companies hoped to appeal to consumers who saw it as an important health benefit. Instead of raising the prices of their fortified foods, manufacturers used irradiation to create a competitive advantage for their products in the marketplace. In 1931, an article in the *New*

York Times noted that irradiated orange juice had a shelf life of seven or eight months, and that General Foods Corporation was already doing further research on irradiation for commercial applications. "Truck gardeners and poultrymen are promised equipment for forcing and producing larger plants and chickens at small cost," the article noted. "Eventually, almost every business and every department of life may be affected."[32]

Frenzied experimentation appeared to be going on nearly everywhere, as rats, chicks, dogs, and other laboratory animals were studied for other elements of dietary deficiency. Commercial laboratories such as those at General Electric were involved, but universities competed as well. University of Cincinnati researchers expanded the idea of "artificial sunshine," claiming they had made it possible to "get your cod-liver oil out of an X-ray tube."[33]

By 1931, people understood the body's need for sunlight and how adding vitamin D to the daily diet could ameliorate the lack of ultraviolet sun or light exposure. "As the air gets more filled with smoke and dirt, and as cities become more crowded and dismal," the *New York Times* noted, "people everywhere, even in the country, enjoy less sunshine." Realizing the sun's importance, "efforts are constantly being made to supply artificially its health-giving elements." Beyond creating vitamin D, by then nicknamed "the sunshine vitamin," it seemed that the entire diet might benefit from ultraviolet exposure in the form of electric light irradiation. Even vitamin D–fortified beer appeared, with the Schlitz company marketing "Sunshine Vitamin D Beer" through World War II.[34]

Irradiation not only added vitamin D, but in 1931 it was discovered to act as an antiseptic, killing bacteria in food, too.

For a time, it appeared that bread, a cheap, universal staple, would be the major product fortified with vitamin D. In 1931, doctors at the Toronto Hospital for Sick Children used simple irradiation technology to add vitamin D to wheat bread. With the addition of irradiated wheat germ, bread could be supplemented with vitamins B and E, as well. The bread tasted fine, and the cost was negligible. Immediately, a US baking firm offered a million dollars to the hospital for the rights to the process. But irradiation of food fell under the control of the Wisconsin Alumni Research Foundation's (WARF) patent of 1924.

Lawsuits for patent infringement popped up everywhere as the burgeoning marketplace of irradiated foods sorted itself out. Even pharmaceutical companies adopted the technology to market vitamin D tonics and supplements made of irradiated oils. Eventually, WARF signed royalty agreements for the right to market Viosterol, a vitamin D supplement, with Parke Davis, Abbott Laboratories, Mead Johnson, E. R. Squibb, and Winthrop Chemical Company.[35]

There was only one food product that chemist Harry Steenbock and WARF refused to allow to be fortified with vitamin D by irradiation: oleomargarine. Margarine manufacturers, the nemesis of the Wisconsin dairy industry, sought to add vitamin D to their product, but the Wisconsin patent holders refused. At the time, margarine's only nutritional claim was based on the addition of vitamin A, done following World War I, and vitamin D would have given it even more status in the marketplace. In 1942 WARF relented, finally selling rights to margarine manufacturers.[36]

TOO MUCH OF A GOOD THING?

While foodstuffs could be irradiated, enriching them with vitamin D, it was a bulky, slow process. Isolating the vitamin element itself and creating an additive made more economic sense. In 1927, the discovery that ergosterol was a form of vitamin D found in plants and fungi was key to moving ahead with a synthetic form of vitamin D that could be taken as a dietary supplement or added to food.[37] Ergosterol, made from irradiated yeast, became a potent form of vitamin D—some claimed it was "a million times as active as average cod liver oil." Although no one really understood it, the remarkable ability of irradiated ergosterol to cure children of rickets—and quickly—made it "one of the most remarkable of specifics," according to one physician. It was a near-miracle therapy. The standard dose of cod liver oil, three teaspoons a day, was too much for a baby yet not enough to cure older children quickly. A few drops of irradiated ergosterol, however, digested easily and worked with alacrity. Hospitals, such as the Hospital for Joint Diseases in New York City, reported dramatic results. Craniotabes, a condition in which an infant's skull softens, cleared up within two weeks. Irradiated ergosterol was remarkable. It was successful. And it was cheap.[38]

While hopes were high that people would "take your daily dose of sunshine as you eat," as one advertisement advised, there was the problem of how much irradiated food or ergosterol doses one should consume. Could a person overdo it? If worried parents gave a child cod liver oil, irradiated foods, *and* light treatments, might they do the youngster harm? No one knew the answer.[39]

Experience soon proved that yes, you could have too much of a good thing. High doses of vitamin D were dangerous, even fatal in some cases. A distinct amount, between too much and too little, was optimal for health and growth. Experimental dosages of ten thousand times the effective dose caused rapid weight loss, emaciation, diarrhea, and eventual death within days in laboratory animals.[40] While the animal experiments were based on huge doses, it still lent caution to how much vitamin D humans should consume. Steenbock found that laboratory animals died when given large amounts of the irradiated ergosterol. "The animal body's tolerance to vitamin D is extremely great," he said. "No ill effects follow the daily consumption of one thousand times as much vitamin D as the minimum amount required to cure rickets." The problem came when ten thousand times the necessary amount was fed to animals, something unlikely if not impossible to happen in normal activity; but an overdose was quite possible if overeager consumers ingested too much.[41]

Besides pinpointing exactly how much vitamin D should be consumed, there was also the problem of standardizing the dosage. By 1930, irradiated ergosterol was being manufactured and sold by a variety of companies (all under the approval of the Wisconsin Alumni Research Foundation), and none of their products were alike. Irradiated ergosterol had no uniform identity: in some cases it was brown and oily, in others it was white and crystalline. Potencies ranged widely with no standardization, as the inexpensive new form of vitamin D was added to tonics, foods, and beverages for health-conscious consumers. Many products were aimed at children, but how could a parent know if her child was getting too little or too much vitamin D?

The Wisconsin Alumni Research Foundation found itself in the middle of the situation and determined a standard for production: the product must be one hundred times as potent as cod liver oil. The suggested daily dose for children was recognized as 8 to 10 drops, or 100D, which meant one hundred times the potency of a dose of cod liver oil. For older children and adults, doses of up to twenty drops daily were suggested.[42]

At the close of 1931, scientists at Mead, Johnson and Company in Evansville, Indiana, announced they had successfully synthesized vitamin D as ergosterol in the laboratory using yeast. The Steenbock irradiation process patent at the University of Wisconsin no longer controlled how vitamin D supplementation was made or what food products it could appear in.

A RACE OF SUPERHUMANS?

Sunlight's effect on the body, long misunderstood and mysterious, had been harnessed, patented, commodified, standardized, and prescribed. Nature was under control, or so it seemed. Amid the grim reality of the Great Depression, laboratory breakthroughs in vitamin research promised a better life ahead. "Because the importance of vitamins is now generally recognized," Dr. R. H. Dennett told a *New York Times* reporter, "the world may look forward to seeing the finest children it has ever known." Vitamins were not a passing fad, he emphasized. Stronger, sturdier bodies due to a "vitamin diet" had the potential to produce a "Super-Race." What happened to fresh air, clean food, and sunshine? Those Progressive era public health ideals took a backseat as modern synthetic vitamins began to appear on store shelves.[43]

Chapter Four

SUNLIGHT AS NUTRIENT

Through technology, sunlight could be duplicated with electric lightbulbs, substituting man-made dietary vitamin D for sunlight exposure. But "making" sunshine was the easy part. Figuring out how sunlight affects the body has taken much longer.

For most people today, vitamin D is just another of the assorted nutrients we can pick and choose from the drugstore shelf. Like the rest of the vitamins that caught the nation's attention in the 1920s and 1930s, it was eventually manufactured, widely available, and that seemed the end of the story. While some of the vitamins and their activity in the body were easy to identify and define, vitamin D turned out to be more complex. It's different from other nutrients that are found only in food because it's a nutrient our bodies create naturally if we get enough sunlight.

Dr. Reinhold Vieth, director of the Bone and Mineral Laboratory, Department of Pathology and Laboratory Medicine at Mount Sinai Hospital in Toronto, points out: "The notion that true nutrients may be available only from foods is a misconception; vitamin D, like niacin, is a vitamin that can be acquired without eating it." Niacin is made in small amounts in the body from the amino acid tryptophan, found in foods from animal sources. Vitamin D, made in the skin from sunlight, can be absorbed through the digestive system as well. It's available, but scarce, in the food supply, and historically people have relied on sunshine to spark chemical activity within the human body. Only in the past eighty years have we figured out how to supplement sunshine—a trick vital for survival due to what Vieth calls "the biological consequences of modern life."[1]

Vitamin D is formed in the skin when ultraviolet light opens up the B-ring of 7-dehydrocholesterol to form previtamin D (cholecalciferol) in the skin. It moves to the liver where it's converted into 25-hydroxyvitamin D, termed

25(OH)D, or calcidiol. Carried by the bloodstream, 25(OH)D moves to the kidney and other tissues where it is converted into 1,25-dihydroxyvitamin D, also called calcitriol, or D_3. Vitamin D is actually a steroid with one of its rings disrupted, often referred to as a prehormone. Other steroid hormones include testosterone, estradiol (estrogen), and cortisol (for normal response to stress).[2] They are some of the most powerful and essential elements in the body.

It wasn't until the mid-1970s that researchers realized D_3 (cholecalciferol) is produced initially in the skin by UV radiation and that it isn't simply a nutrient but a hormone that causes metabolic changes in the body. Vitamin D moves and regulates calcium and phosphorus through the bloodstream in a complicated process that is still not completely understood.[3] New research is published monthly from a wide spectrum of sciences; bone specialists, endocrinologists, nutritionists, dermatologists, and biochemists are only some of the fields concerned with vitamin D's complex actions in the body.

VITAMIN D THROUGH THE DIGESTIVE SYSTEM

Our bodies are designed to absorb vitamin D from sunlight but we also make use of its nutritional benefits through the digestive system. Whether from skin or the digestive system, vitamin D is inactive when it enters the body and must be utilized in a biologically active form. This occurs in the kidneys, liver, and many other body tissues. An interesting way to look at the puzzle behind humans' complex system of getting vitamin D is to examine animals. Most vertebrates need vitamin D to absorb calcium for bone health, just as we do, and they make it on their body surface: fur, feathers, and skin all create the precursor, or preliminary chemical stage that eventually results in vitamin D when they expose themselves to ultraviolet radiation from sunlight. Birds and fur-bearing animals get their natural vitamin D by grooming themselves with their beaks and tongues, thereby licking the body oils laden with this vitamin D precursor off their fur and feathers. Chickens and livestock reared entirely indoors away from natural sunlight need to have vitamin D supplements added to their feed if they are to grow and thrive because they're unable to make it on their body surface without sunlight. Animals without fur or feathers, such as pigs and humans, make their vitamin D directly through the skin—no body licking required. Vitamin D can be extracted from UV-exposed human sweat, too.[4]

Normally, rays from the sun are absorbed by the skin and induce conversion of 7-dehydrocholesterol into vitamin D_3 (cholecalciferol), but if enough dietary vitamin D is consumed from food sources, the process begins in the intestine. Either way, (cholecalciferol) moves to the liver, where it's changed to a form of the vitamin known as 25(OH)D, and circulates in the bloodstream or is stored in fat cells until needed. The parathyroid gland (attached to the thyroid) releases parathyroid hormone, which regulates the body's use of the minerals calcium, magnesium, and phosphate in the bloodstream by alerting the liver to send vitamin D to the kidney, where it's converted into calcitriol and is sent out to tissues. Once activated as calcitriol, vitamin D enters the nucleus of a cell, where it begins a series of interactions that control more than 1,000 genes in tissues throughout the body. This elaborate process has received an enormous amount of research—over five thousand scientific papers have addressed the subject—and the complexity is still being unraveled.[5]

CLARIFYING TERMS

Calcidiol (the inactive circulating vitamin D), calcitriol (the active form of vitamin D), cholecalciferol (vitamin D_3), ergocalciferol (vitamin D_2)—the terms are mind-boggling, and indeed, some researchers and physicians stumble over them, this author included. To make it less confusing to the layperson, this book will use terms vitamin D and cholecalciferol interchangeably at times. When referring to supplements, the specific terms D_3 or D_2 will be used. While vitamin D acts as a hormone in the body, it can be ingested as a supplement or in food, wending its way to the liver via the digestive system rather than through the bloodstream from the skin. Vitamin D expert Reinhold Vieth makes an excellent point by arguing that vitamin D should be identified as a nutrient—not a hormone—because the "misconception that Vitamin D is a hormone creates a situation where people who may benefit from Vitamin D will avoid it along with what many regard as the unnecessary use of hormones."[6] It's a nutrient, but one that can nourish the body by entering through the skin as well as the digestive system.

ROLE IN BONE BUILDING

Vitamin D is vital for building and repairing bones, but it doesn't actually build bones; it regulates and transports the calcium and phosphorus needed for the process. When calcium and phosphorus are available in adequate amounts due to vitamin D, mineralization of bone takes place, which maintains its strength. In adults, bones are continually remodeling; new bone cells replace discarded ones so that the skeleton renews itself (achieves bone cell replacement) every seven years. In adults, bones aren't growing longer anymore, but they continue to remodel and create fresh cells. If adequate D levels aren't readily available to the bones, collagen in bone doesn't mineralize, thereby making adult bones soft (like those of young children) or weak and prone to fracture. In growing children, low D levels result in failure of bones to mineralize. As they grow, children's bones then enlarge without adequate minerals and weight-bearing legs and spine bend out of shape; for instance, girls' pelvic bones fail to form properly. In babies, the fontanel, or soft spot on the skull, grows together more slowly than normal, while teeth develop poorly and come in later. Low calcium levels in infants can also lead to tetany (spasms of face, hands, and feet) and seizures.[7]

VITAMIN D AND TUMOR GROWTH

Vitamin D also regulates the proliferating cells (those that are dividing rapidly), which is an important aspect of growth in young children. But because uncontrolled proliferation of cells is also how cancer tumors grow and spread, researchers are studying the role vitamin D plays in regulating the growth of cells through what's called cell differentiation. Cell differentiation results in the specialization of cells for specific functions, decreasing simple proliferation. Cells devote themselves to targeted activities and no longer simply reproduce by cell division. Vitamin D plays a role in stopping that uncontrolled reproduction of cells (proliferation), which is associated with diseases like cancer, and directs cells toward specific activities (differentiation). Inadequate amounts of vitamin D may allow proliferation, and cancer, because the cells lack adequate regulating mechanisms to direct them toward specific activities.

REGULATING THE IMMUNE SYSTEM

Vitamin D is also necessary in regulating the immune system and may enhance immunity and inhibit autoimmunity—diseases in which the body destroys its own cells, such as multiple sclerosis and rheumatoid arthritis. This area offers the greatest potential for research, because both vitamin D levels and melatonin levels have been linked to immunity, as will be discussed later in this book. Melatonin, a hormone produced in the brain's pineal gland, regulates the body's response to lightness and darkness. Sunlight has a well-established effect on the immune system, which might explain seasonal epidemics, such as influenza, which often occur in winter in the colder climates when body levels are low. Also, levels of both appear to decline in adulthood, particularly for women, making the immune system less protective and generating many diseases common in advanced years.[8]

INSULIN ACTIVITY

Vitamin D activity regulates insulin, the hormone created in the pancreas to control the level of sugar in the body. Some results suggest that low D levels in humans may affect insulin and glucose activity leading to both type 1 and type 2 diabetes. Type 1 diabetes, often appearing in infancy or childhood, and thought to be genetically caused, has been linked to low prenatal levels of vitamin D in the mother and low levels in childhood. Studies in Finland and Italy have found that supplementation during pregnancy and infancy may prevent the development of type 1 diabetes.[9] The risk of developing type 2 (non-insulin) diabetes, often appearing in middle-age adults, is reduced for those people with adequate vitamin D levels. In one study, people with highest levels reduced their risk for developing type 2 diabetes by 40 percent.[10]

MULTIPLE CHRONIC DISEASES LINKED TO VITAMIN D DEFICIENCY

Because D acts by enabling genes to "turn on" proteins and enzymes crucial to hundreds of tissues in the body, the lack of D is implicated in a multitude of chronic diseases; in fact, an avalanche of new research suggests that most chronic disease conditions are probably linked to low levels of vitamin D.[11] For some conditions, years of research supports the link to vitamin D deficiency, but for others the research is just beginning. Because vitamin D works in such complex ways within the body, it's still unclear how it affects some diseases. In some cases it appears to act as a preventive, while for others it may only be effective to reduce the symptoms of the chronic disease.

Here's a short laundry list of some disease conditions now believed to be related to low vitamin D levels:

- Autoimmune diseases (those affecting the immune system)
- Cancer: breast, prostate, colon, skin
- Cardiovascular disease
- Chronic low-back pain
- Depression
- Diabetes type 1 and 2
- Epilepsy
- Fibromyalgia
- Hypertension
- Inflammatory bowel disease
- Lupus erythematosus
- Migraine headaches
- Multiple sclerosis
- Musculoskeletal pain
- Osteoarthritis
- Osteomalacia
- Osteoporosis
- Periodontal disease
- Polycystic ovary syndrome
- Rheumatoid arthritis
- Rickets
- Tetany

Researchers are also looking at vitamin D's impact on developing premenstrual syndrome, schizophrenia, and even male baldness. It seems there are few body systems untouched by the importance of sunlight.

BLOOD TESTS TO ASSESS VITAMIN D LEVELS IN THE BODY

If adequate levels of vitamin D in the body are so crucial, how do we know how much our body has stored? Just as our knowledge of how much sunshine we really need to receive is still unclear, it's also difficult to figure out how much vitamin D our body contains. Vitamin D can be circulating in the blood, stored in the liver and fat cells, or active within targeted cells; there's no technique for measuring it all at once. In fact, there are two vitamin D tests; the 25(OH)D test measures the level of calcidiol (the inactive form) that is circulating in the bloodstream. This is the main form of vitamin D stored in the body. About 99 percent of the vitamin D in the blood is in the form of calcidiol. The other test, the 25-hydroxy-vitamin D test, measures the amount of calcidiol the kidney converts into active calcitriol, by assessing the level of calcitriol in the blood. Experts disagree over which test is better, but the 25(OH)D test for calcidiol is most commonly used.

Like everything else surrounding vitamin D, interpreting test results is complicated, too. The ideal levels for vitamin D status in the blood are debatable and no solid figures are accepted as cut-offs for deficiency or sufficiency levels. Lab reference ranges are based on average values for healthy groups tested rather than optimal levels based on solid research data. Generally, 25(OH)D levels below 20-25 nmol/L (nanomoles/liter) indicate severe deficiency—at that level it's very likely you already have rickets or osteomalacia (weakening bones). A level of 50 nmol/L had been considered reasonably healthy, but new research indicates values should be approximately 80 nmol/L for optimal function. Ideal vitamin D levels from the 25-hydroxy-vitamin D test should be between 45 and 50 ng/ml, or 115 to 128 nmol/L.[12]

OPTIMAL LEVELS

Just as it's difficult to determine how much vitamin D we have in our body, experts don't agree on how much vitamin D we should carry in the bloodstream, nor do they agree on how often we should test our blood levels for the hormone. As Dr. John Cannell, Vitamin D Council director, explains: "How much vitamin D you need varies with age, body weight, percent of body fat, [geographic] latitude, skin coloration, season of the year, use of sun block, individual variation in sun exposure, and—probably—how ill you are. As a general rule, old people need more than young people, big people need more than little people, fat people need more than skinny people, northern people need more than southern people, dark-skinned people need more than fair skinned people, winter people need more than summer people, sun block lovers need more than sun block haters, sun-phobes need more than sun worshipers, and ill people may need more than well people."[13]

It's probably the most variable nutrient or health component in the body and the easiest to replenish. The level in the blood can be increased by using supplements or by sunlight exposure and is usually higher during summer months and lower during winter, as the body uses up its stores of vitamin D held in fat cells. Studies indicate that adults who live in temperate latitudes, such as North America, need to intake at least 2,000 IU (International Units) of vitamin D per day to achieve 25(OH)D levels of at least 80 nmol/L. If you intend to supplement your sunshine exposure by taking vitamin D supplements, be sure to have a blood test before you begin and use the advice of a nutritionist or physician. While the body can never absorb too much D from sunshine, because the body turns off the process of absorbing ultraviolet radiation through the skin when enough has been absorbed, it's possible to ingest too much via supplementation. That's because vitamin D, a fat-soluble vitamin, is stored in our fat cells and ingesting too much through the digestive system can be harmful because there's no automatic shutoff through that route of absorbing vitamin D.

TOO MUCH VITAMIN D?

Because it's a fat-soluble nutrient and stored in the body, it's possible to have too much vitamin D in the body. While such conditions seldom occur, as people begin dosing themselves with vitamin D_3 (cholecalciferol) available now as a supplement, it could potentially occur. Vitamin D toxicity (hypervitaminosis D) causes very high levels of calcium in the blood, which can harm bones, cause kidney stones, and lead to calcification of the heart and kidneys. The Food and Nutrition Board at the Institute of Medicine set an upper limit of 2,000 IU/day (50 micrograms/day) for children and adults. Some recent research suggests such a limit is too low and that healthy people can safely take

10,000 IU/day, but there isn't a consensus within the medical community yet to support that high level.[14]

Therapeutic doses may be much higher in order to attain results. In a Wisconsin study done in 2008, nursing home residents were given 50,000 IU of vitamin D_2 (ergocalciferol) three times a week for four weeks. By that time their vitamin D blood levels were normal. No ill effects were observed, even on such high doses. Some researchers suggest we may need much higher levels than recognized if taking vitamin D in supplement form. With age, the ability to absorb or metabolize vitamin D, whether from sunlight or supplement, drops, although our need for vitamin D remains constant.[15]

Overdoses do occur, such as one in Italy where a sixty-two-year-old man and his fifty-five-year-old wife were given a series of injections of vitamin D by their physician, inadvertently overdosing them with large amounts of vitamin D. They were hospitalized and their blood tested at over 150 ng/mL (normal range is 16 to 74 ng/mL). X-rays showed the man had calcification of the arteries and muscles, and both had kidney failure due to the overdose of vitamin D. Their condition improved after treatment, which included drinking lots of water, and taking furosemide and prednisone to flush the vitamin D from the body. While cases like this are thankfully not widespread, it indicates a need to use caution when dosing with large amounts of supplemental vitamin D.[16]

PROBLEMS WITH FOOD FORTIFICATION

Because there's a risk of getting too much vitamin D, fortifying foods with additional vitamin D is controversial. In Canada vitamin D_3 fortification of milk and margarine is required by law; in the United States it is legally allowed to be added to several foods but is generally added only to fluid milk. Federal law does not require vitamin D fortification of milk unless the label claims it to be fortified. Also, federal regulations stipulate that when milkfat is removed from milk (such as skim milk and 2% milk), vitamin A must be added back to milk because it was originally in whole milk. Vitamin manufacturers package vitamins A and D together, so most dairy processors add the two together, although there is no requirement to add vitamin D back to milk because it didn't exist there in the first place. Vitamin D supplementation does add value to milk, making it even more nutritious, and advertisers once promoted it as "liquid sunshine." Adding vitamin D to milk is logical because it helps the body utilize the minerals milk contains, particularly calcium and magnesium.

Many people wrongly assume that all dairy products are sources of vitamin D, but this is not true. Because other dairy products, such as cottage cheese, cheese, ice cream, and yogurts are not supplemented, consumers are often led astray, consuming plenty of dairy to get their calcium but failing to consume enough D to make it effective within the body. Cold cereals are often fortified with vitamin D and when consumed with milk they gain the added fortification from the milk. Other food products, such as juices, may be fortified with vitamin D, but one needs to read the label to be sure because inconsistencies abound.

Studies suggest that current US/Canadian food fortification programs aren't all that successful in preventing inadequate vitamin D levels, especially among people who need increased amounts (due to having darker skin pigment or low metabolism levels) and during winter months. Although adding vitamin D to milk seemed logical, it has not been the best source of the vitamin for many people. Many adults have difficulty digesting milk (many are lactose intolerant—meaning they can't ingest the lactic acid in milk) or don't like the taste. African Americans, who have the greatest need for vitamin D, have the lowest intake from fortified food and dairy products.[17] Children and teens, those who most need vitamin D and calcium for growing bones, opt for more soda pop and sugared fruit juices than milk. Teen girls and weight-conscious women avoid drinking milk with meals as a way to stay slim since they perceive milk as high in fat. Also a number of immigrant cultures in the United States, such as Southwest Asians, didn't consume milk as part of their traditional diet and haven't adopted it here; nor are they eating the traditional food sources of calcium found in their homeland. Lacking sunlight and traditional sources of calcium such as bone broths, figs, or seafood, immigrant groups don't get the vitamin D or calcium they need.

Vegetarians who strictly limit intake of animal-based foods may also find it difficult to get adequate vitamin D and calcium levels. Anyone pursuing a vegan diet (absolutely no animal-based foods) should be fully aware of what nutrients they are getting and be sure to maintain adequate vitamin D levels, whether from supplements or sunshine.

THE SUPPLEMENT SOLUTION?

For most people who lead modern active lives, supplements have replaced sunlight as a source of vitamin D. For most people, taking a synthetic supplement makes a lot of sense because food sources are inconsistent and these individuals seldom get into the sun for extended periods of time. And supplements are an important source of vitamin D as people age because skin thickness and ability to absorb and create vitamin D declines over time. One study found twenty-year-olds make twice the amount of vitamin D in their skin from sun exposure as those aged sixty-eight to eighty years. The amount of melanin in the skin acts as a natural sunscreen, too, meaning people with darker pigmented skin need to spend more time in the sun to create adequate amounts of vitamin D.[18]

Vitamin D as a vitamin supplement has its roots in cod liver oil, the original folk supplement we discussed in chapter 3. Vitamins, hormones, and medications are measured in IU, or International Units, based upon their biological activity. The measurement is unique to each substance, and there's no correlation between various substances. One IU of vitamin D does not compare to one IU of anything else. The recommended amount of vitamin D, or "International Units" (IU) set as the Recommended Dietary Allowance (RDA) for adults, is based on the amount of vitamin D activity in cod liver oil. In 1941, when the RDA for vitamin D was established, it was set at 400 IU because that was equal to a teaspoon of cod liver oil—the amount found necessary to keep infants from developing rickets.[19]

Vitamin D supplements are inexpensive and widely available, but like the rest of vitamin D, the story is complex. Vitamin D comes in two forms: D_2, or ergosterol, made by irradiating yeast or plant sterols with UV lights; and D_3, or cholecalciferol, made by irradiating skin with UV light. They are both forms of vitamin D, with slightly different chemical bonds. Both are metabolized within the body from supplements and have been considered equally effective. Some studies show vitamin D_3 raises blood levels of vitamin D more effectively than D_2, but more research needs to be done.

In 1937, German scientists A. Windaus and F. Bock first developed D_3 by irradiating the skin of pigs. Ultraviolet light exposure activates vitamin D in skin, feathers, hair, or wool, as well as in foods of animal origin, such as butter and fish oils.[20]

It was a departure from Steenbock's method of irradiating foods to fortify them, making vitamin D in much the same way our skin does when exposed to sunlight. Today, D_3 is manufactured under a patented process held by the chemical company Philips-Duphar. They began making synthetic vitamin D by irradiating yeasts to make and sell vitamin D–enriched chocolate candy in the 1920s. Years later they developed a process for creating vitamin D by irradiating sea mussels. While the exact process in today's D_3 remains a trade secret, it involves treating the cholesterol in lanolin from sheep's wool with ultraviolet light. When stimulated by ultraviolet light, the lipid cells in the wool create cholecalciferol, which is extracted from the wool with chemicals and dried into a white crystalline form that can be added to foods or supplements.

A RAT POISON?

Philips-Duphar, a firm based in the Netherlands and currently owned by Solvay Pharmaceuticals, is the world's source for synthetic cholecalciferol (vitamin D_3). They make a variety of chemical compounds, including herbicides, insecticides, and pharmaceuticals. Their factories in India process some of the cholecalciferol as well. In the United States, the Bell Laboratory plant in Madison, Wisconsin, formulates the Philips-Duphar cholecalciferol into a very effective rodenticide, sold as Quintox. In that form, it is recognized by the United States Department of Agriculture as an allowable rodenticide on certified organic farms. As a rat poison, it's applied around the base of walls or inside transport vehicles (airplanes, trains, trucks) to kill rats and mice. It's so effective that rats need ingest only one dose before they die.

Cholecalciferol in large amounts causes calcification of the blood vessels, the heart muscle, and eventually other organs, leading to heart failure and death. Researchers tried the stuff on primates, likely to see how humans would react to the poison, and found apes died about two months after being given small doses for thirty days. Humans respond the same way, showing symptoms of cholecalciferol poisoning as follows:

- Anorexia
- Elevated blood pressure
- Heart palpitations
- High concentration of calcium in the blood

- Itchiness
- Lethargy and muscle weakness
- Nausea and vomiting
- Nervousness

Yet by the time symptoms of too much cholecalciferol are observed, the heart muscle has been damaged beyond repair. Postmortem examination reveals calcification in the kidneys, liver, lungs, blood vessels, and heart.[21]

Cholecalciferol is difficult to expel from the body; it's fat soluble and stays in fat cells for weeks, so any treatment for overdosing takes time as the body must use up the stored amounts in order to detoxify. While individuals respond differently to cholecalciferol poisoning, treatments suggested for humans include magnesium sulphate, cortisone, and calcitonin. Anyone suspected to have ingested too much cholecalciferol should see a physician for testing and treatment.

Veterinarians have found prednisone given every twelve hours orally to be successful in saving animals accidentally sickened by cholecalciferol rat poison. Prednisone halts the action of too much cholecalciferol because it decreases calcium concentrations in the body by preventing bones from utilizing calcium, preventing calcium absorption in the intestines, and increasing the amount of calcium excreted by the kidneys. Interestingly, those very actions show how drugs like prednisone create havoc in the normal healthy body by preventing the body from using calcium and vitamin D in normal bone processes. If one takes prednisone regularly, efforts should be made to replenish the vitamin D it flushes from the body.[22]

HOW MUCH IS TOO MUCH?

While cholecalciferol poisoning may be a concern for pet owners whose animal accidentally eats rat poison, it's quite likely that enthusiastic individuals may respond to promotions from vitamin D supplement makers and overdose themselves on cholecalciferol. Because there have been so few cases of overdose in humans and human research can't really be done, experts vary in what they consider to be levels of toxicity. The Linus Pauling Institute, located at Oregon State University, points to a consumption of 10,000 IU daily over a period of months as possibly too much to ingest. Less conservative estimates believe that to achieve levels of concern, one would need to ingest levels of 100,000 IU/day over several months.

Other countries use megadoses of cholecalciferol as a therapeutic and a preventative (most do not fortify food with cholecalciferol). Massive doses of vitamin D are used in Europe to prevent hip fracture in the elderly. Annual injections of up to 150,000 IU or oral supplementation every four months of 100,000 IU have no side effects.

Overdoses seldom occur or are undiagnosed, and it's not clear how dangerous too much vitamin D can actually be. A recent case of accidental overdose of ergocalciferol (the D_2 form of the vitamin) occurred when a mother gave her thirty-two-pound son too much of a liquid preparation made in Latin America. Instead of giving one drop (2,500 IU) per day, the amount the directions stated for adult dosage, the mother gave one bottle daily for four days: 2,400,000 IU in all. The child developed abdominal pain, high blood pressure, and high blood calcium levels, but he recovered once the diagnosis was made.[23]

Regardless the isolated incidents of vitamin D overdose, it's extremely rare and not likely to occur when individuals are taking amounts prescribed by physicians or daily supplements within normal limits. Like anything else, vitamin D can be problematic when taken in massive amounts—just as drinking too much water can cause deadly water intoxication.

SUNLIGHT IS SAFEST

Exposure to sunlight, however, never results in an overdose of vitamin D. The body simply stops creating vitamin D when levels are maximized. The concentration of previtamin D in the skin reaches equilibrium in white skin within twenty minutes of ultraviolet exposure and stops making the previtamin form of vitamin D. Pigmented skin can take three to six times longer to reach equilibrium concentration of previtamin D in the skin. Skin pigment doesn't affect the amount of vitamin D that can be obtained through sunshine, it just takes longer to achieve adequate levels. Aging, too, reduces the capacity for vitamin D production in the skin. After skin exposure, the initial form of previtamin circulates in the bloodstream, is then converted to vitamin D in the liver and kidney, and is stored until needed by the body. Moderation is necessary, however, because overexposure leads to sunburn, skin damage, and concerns about developing skin cancer.[24]

VITAMIN D ANALOGS

New research reveals that vitamin D does much more than moderate calcium and phosphorus absorption in the body; it has effects on cell differentiation and proliferation and can modulate immune responses and central nervous system functioning. It also acts as a cancer preventive because it can switch off the ability of cells to multiply and spread. Vitamin D analogs—chemical structures that duplicate the naturally occurring form of the vitamin—are under development and offer potential for treatment for several diseases because they can be manipulated to eliminate the molecular composition that makes large doses of vitamin D toxic. If analogs, or vitamin D drugs, can be created that eliminate particular unwanted actions—such as calcium regulation—while maintaining the ability to shut down tumor growth, medications could be created to intervene in a wide variety of cell activities.

Active vitamin D_2 and D_3 analogs are under development as therapies for cancer tumors and hyperparathyroidism (excess production of parathyroid hormone). D_2 made by irradiating yeast with UV light has been successful in controlling cell proliferation in the lab. Because cancer tumors rely on rapidly growing cells, it may be a way to halt cancer in its tracks. Vitamin D regulates parathyroid growth and parathyroid hormone production, stimulates activity in the pancreas (the insulin-producing organ), and bolsters the immune system, making a wide variety of analogs potentially valuable.

TOPICAL VITAMIN D

Parents who have used the commercial preparation A & D Ointment for their baby's diaper rash know how effective the topical application of vitamins (in this case, A and D) can be. While cod liver oil is a component of that particular commercial ointment, there are other forms of vitamin D that are prescription-only medications to be applied to the skin. Calcipotriene and tacalcitol are vitamin D analogs, synthesized matches (almost) to actual vitamin D. Calcipotriene is sold as Dovonex ointment, prescribed by dermatologists for psoriasis and skin problems. It appears to slow excessive growth of skin cells; however, the exact mechanism of action is unknown. Tacalcitol, another vitamin D analog, binds to the keratinocyte (a type of skin cell) vitamin D receptor in the same manner as vitamin D. It acts by normalizing cell growth and development in the skin. In cases of psoriasis, it prevents the excessive growth rate of skin cells that leads to scaling of the skin.

ELUSIVE NATURAL SOURCES

If you don't drink milk (which is fortified) and are uncomfortable ingesting synthetic cholecalciferol as a supplement, where do you get D? There aren't many natural food sources of vitamin D. Oily fish, such as herring, sardines (eat the bones, too, for the calcium), tuna, mackerel, trout, and salmon, cod liver oil, and sun-dried mushrooms are the best natural sources other than sunlight. None are very common in today's Western diet. Traditional fatty-fish foods provided plenty of vitamin D along with healthy fats, but we simply don't eat much oily fish despite the health benefits. Economics, our fast-food culture, worries about depletion due to overfishing, and mercury contamination all push consumers to avoid oily fish dishes that were mainstays of most traditional diets.

Molje—made from cod meat, cod liver oil, fish roe (eggs), and boiled potatoes, dripping with butter and egg sauce—is a traditional Norwegian winter food that provides lots of vitamin D. In a study conducted at Skervoy, Norway (latitude 70 degrees north), volunteers ate three molje meals then were given blood tests for vitamin D levels. The three meals provided about fifty-four times the recommended daily dose of vitamin D. Norwegians who ate frequent molje meals during winter sustained satisfactory vitamin D levels, despite the long "vitamin D winter" experienced at far northern latitudes. Oily fish, fish liver, organ meats, insects, and other animal sources of vitamin D were commonly eaten in the past as part of indigenous traditional diets for most people of the world. Butterfat, egg yolks, and fat from poultry are all sources of vitamin D if the animals are raised on green grass pastures. Today, processed foods have replaced many of the foods people once relied on, making it difficult to remain healthy during long winters in northern locales.[25]

A chart from the National Institutes of Health (NIH) lists some of the most commonly consumed sources in the United States. But, the choices are limited, so using food alone as a source for natural vitamin D is extremely difficult. There are also wide variations in the amount of vitamin D in foods depending upon their source and variety. The NIH figures don't take into account whether the salmon tested is farmed or wild, nor do they address the other health problems inherent in their list of suggested food sources for vitamin D. Oily fish, a good source of vitamin D, would have to be consumed at least daily, along with other sources, to reach the suggested threshold of 400 IU intake. Such fish have been ruled too dangerous to consume more than once a week because they contain high levels of mercury and other toxic contaminants. That leaves chicken eggs, which contain some D, but would anyone relish eating seventeen eggs a day to get enough vitamin D? Every day? Or, twenty-five ounces of Swiss cheese? Every day? You could try cereals and milk, but the cereal would drain vitamin D levels (recall May Mellanby's work and the "cereal factor" found in phytic acid, in chapter 3).

Food Sources of Vitamin D

Selected food sources of vitamin D based on a recommended daily allowance of 400 IU of vitamin D for adults age fifty and over from the NIH Office of Dietary Supplements:

Food	International Units (IU) per serving	Percent Daily Value
Cod liver oil, 1 tbsp.	1,360	340
Salmon, cooked 3 1/2 oz.	360	90
Mackerel, cooked 3 1/2 oz.	345	90
Tuna fish, canned in oil, 3 oz.	200	50
Sardines, canned in oil, drained, 1 3/4 oz.	250	70
Milk, nonfat, reduced fat, and whole, vitamin D fortified, 1 cup	98	25

Margarine, fortified, 1 tbsp.	60	15
Pudding, prepared from mix and made with vitamin D fortified milk, 1/2 cup	50	10
Ready-to-eat cereals fortified with 10% of the DV for vitamin D, 3/4 cup to 1 cup servings (servings vary according to the brand)	40	10
Egg, 1 whole (vitamin D is found in egg yolk)	20	6
Liver, beef, cooked, 3 1/2 oz.	15	4
Cheese, Swiss, 1 oz.	12	4

For foods not listed in this table, please refer to the US Department of Agriculture's Nutrient Database Web site:
http://www.nal.usda.gov/fnic/cgi-bin/nut_search.pl.
For another source that cites different amounts of vitamin D in the same foods, see "Provisional Table on the Vitamin D Content of Foods," from the Human Nutrition Service of the USDA, HNIS/PT-108.

THE COD FISHERY

Since cod liver oil has traditionally been the best alternative to sunlight as a source of vitamin D, it's important to look at what's happening to cod. In the 1980s, overfishing in the North Atlantic caused codfish stocks to dwindle to near exhaustion. The cods' food source, herring, mackerel, and menhaden, had already been in decline a decade earlier due to overfishing. The Atlantic supply of cod is so low governments have agreed to prohibit fishing. In 1992, data assembled by the United Nations Food and Agriculture Organization identified Atlantic codfish as depleted or overfished. Northern Atlantic and Arctic cod, the kind from which cod liver oil is obtained, are still being fished, however, in spite of warnings by scientists in Denmark that there will soon be no cod to argue over.[26]

Besides worrying that cod may disappear, there is additional fear that cod fish oil might be contaminated with heavy metals. Mercury, selenium, and other toxins have been found in fish, leading the United States government to warn against consuming too much fish in the diet, which may overload the body with toxins. While fish oils in general should be scrutinized because many fatty fish contain contaminants, cod seem to have escaped the pollutants. Lab tests on cod liver oil have found very low levels of contaminants. Still, while cod liver oil is a lifesaver right now, we don't have any guarantee that it will remain available and unpolluted. Other fish oils, while excellent sources of omega-3 fatty acids, may or may not contain adequate amounts of vitamin D, depending upon the fish used.[27]

Cod liver oil may also be problematic because it contains high amounts of vitamin A, another fat-soluble nutrient that is stored in the body. Vitamins A and D have similar receptors in the cell nucleus and too much A in the cell can block levels of D, eventually affecting a person's calcium uptake because there's not enough D to regulate the calcium. For that reason, ingesting more than 1400 mg of vitamin A daily has been linked to an increase in hip fractures. So, even with adequate vitamin D and calcium in the diet, too much vitamin A can prevent vitamin D from making the calcium available.

MUSHROOM RESEARCH

The cod fishery is declining. Vitamin D_3 added to fortify skim milk often dissipates because the milk fat isn't there to store it. Processed cholecalciferol supplements seem unnatural and may not be available. Yet, if we live in northern latitudes, vitamin D deficiency is rampant. If we can't get enough sun, what can we do?

In the future, dried mushrooms, of all things, may prove the best choice for garnering vitamin D in a healthful, easy, and inexpensive manner. Dried mushrooms seem as odd as cod livers as an alternative to sunshine for humans, yet, for centuries, people in Southeast Asia and China have added handfuls of dried mushrooms to meals, unknowingly garnering significant amounts of vitamin D, along with other nutrients found in mushrooms.

Mushrooms naturally contain some vitamin D, in the form of D_2, the plant form of ergosterol. When exposed to sunlight, however, fresh mushrooms react like human skin—they create their own vitamin D. That vitamin D is in the form of ergosterol, the plant form of vitamin D and the form used in prescription doses of the vitamin. (Cholecalciferol, D_3, is the form added to milk and found in over-the-counter supplements.) While mushrooms, contain vitamin D, no one really knew whether humans could absorb it until researchers in Finland tested a group of volunteers who consumed wild mushrooms. The wild mushrooms used, *Cantharellus tubaeformis*, were purchased in autumn, then blended and homogenized with broth and fed to the study participants during January when no sunlight could affect results. A test group given vitamin D supplements instead of mushrooms showed similar blood level rise, while a the control group, given neither mushrooms nor supplement, remained low.[28]

Paul Stamets, a mycologist (fungi specialist) on the Olympic Peninsula of Washington State, has been engaged in research on these remarkable plants for decades. Since the 1960s, *Basidiomycetes* mushrooms have been known to show antitumor action and have shown potential for cancer prevention and treatment. Stamets followed up this work by examining how levels of vitamin D in mushrooms affect their anticancer activity and came up with amazing results. Dried forms of reishi, shiitake, and maitake mushrooms naturally contain some vitamin D; in levels of 6 (for reishi), 134 (for shiitake), and 460 IU per 100 grams (for maitake). When Stamets dried mushrooms outdoors for six to eight hours in natural sunlight, however, he discovered that the amounts increased to a whopping 2760 IU, 21,400 IU, and 31,900 IU of vitamin D per 100 grams, respectively, for the dried mushroom, an incredible amount of vitamin D available from a naturally sun-dried plant source.[29]

His work challenges the long-held USDA claim that common button mushrooms contain 76 IU of vitamin D per 100 grams; or that dried shiitake mushrooms contain 1550 IU per 100 grams. Stamets's findings throw a kink in all dietary work done involving mushrooms in the past because nutritionists relied on USDA data, which is clearly inaccurate. He also opened the door to studying vitamin D action in the body and how to use mushrooms as alternative supplements to chemically derived cholecalciferol.

Sun-dried (or artificially UV treated) mushrooms provide a clear alternative to dangerous supplements of cholecalciferol, manufactured by chemical companies. Sun-dried mushrooms can't be consumed in levels that endanger health, like cholecalciferol can. The mushroom source of vitamin D is ergocalciferol, a plant sterol, which the body processes into the active form of vitamin D, cholecalciferol. When there's plenty of cholecalciferol (D_3) in the body's stores, it shuts down processing any more from ergocalciferol.

CONTAMINANTS CREATE CAUTION

Mushrooms feast on carbons (rotting forest matter) and will also consume petroleum, another form of carbon. They are so effective at "eating" carbon-containing material, they have been used to digest oil spills and other carbon-based contamination. While that's useful in cleaning up waste dumps, it makes them dangerous if they have absorbed the wrong nutrients. Because mushrooms are able to absorb and concentrate heavy metals, if pesticides or fungicides have been used during production or near the farm, they may contain harmful quantities. Stamets suggests buying shiitake mushrooms from certified organic growers whose farms are located in pollution-free or near-pollution-free environments. "The unfortunate truth is that mushrooms are a reflection of the environment in which they are grown," he explains. "If the air and land are polluted, the mushrooms grown there will be too."[30]

In 2006, the Food and Drug Administration funded research jointly with the Mushroom Council and found that by using artificial ultraviolet light, Stamets's findings could be applied to mushrooms on an industrial scale. They found that a standard serving size of white button mushrooms, exposed to ultraviolet light/sunlight for five minutes, pushed the vitamin D_2 level to 3476 IU, or 869 percent of the recommended daily intake of vitamin D. In 2006, a Swiss study found that substantial amounts of vitamin D (ergosterol) could be generated through UV light application to most commercial mushrooms: white and brown button, portabella, shiitake, oyster, chanterelles, and king bolete.[31]

Sun-dried or irradiated, mushrooms are an inexpensive, appealing, and digestible way to increase vitamin D levels for everyone, including vegetarian or lactose-intolerant people. Currently, fresh irradiated mushrooms are available from Monterey Mushrooms and Dole, and the market is expected to expand once consumers are aware of the benefits of vitamin D_2 enhancement. You can increase the vitamin D level of fresh mushrooms for yourself by placing them in direct sunlight for five to ten minutes before eating. Or you can preserve them for long winter soups and stews by slicing fresh mushrooms and sun drying them completely before storing in sealed containers. It doesn't seem to matter whether the mushrooms are consumed raw or cooked; they provide a unique source of valuable vitamin D in levels the body can easily and safely absorb.

VITAMIN D IN BAKERY PRODUCTS

A recent patent on another food source providing extra vitamin D may be useful. Yeast, enriched with vitamin D through a unique process, may soon be on the market, found in bread and other baked goods. Yeast contains ergosterol, which when exposed to ultraviolet light creates vitamin D_2 and is easily absorbed in the digestive system. The patented process to create the vitamin is important because ultraviolet light or sunlight will kill microbes, such as viruses, bacteria, molds, and harmful yeasts. The patented process overcomes UV light's deadly effect on yeasts, while activating the ergosterol it can produce. The yeast is still alive and can be used in baked goods. In the future, vitamin D_2–enriched pizza crust, hamburger buns, and sugar cookies may find their way into northern-latitude diets.

While supplementation through engineering yeast holds potential, simply adding water-soluble vitamin D powder to bread dough seemed to work in one study. Rye bread and wheat bread were enriched with vitamin D_3 (cholecalciferol) and eaten by a test panel of students from Helsinki University. They ate four slices of the enriched bread daily for three weeks in midwinter. The study compared their blood levels of vitamin D with another group eating plain bread and taking vitamin D supplements. The blood levels of vitamin D for both groups were similar.[32]

In the future it appears that enriched foods offer potential for adding vitamin D during winter months. It will be hard to figure out whether you have eaten enough foods to ensure adequate levels—or if you've eaten too much, particularly during sunny summer months, when people would likely continue eating fortified foods while absorbing large amounts of ultraviolet light through their skin from sunshine.

ADEQUATE INTAKE

Although research now shows that several foods can be enriched with added vitamin D and that the nutrient is absorbed through the digestive system, eating vitamin D may not be a complete solution. The problem with adding vitamin D to foods is that there's no way to ensure how much is consumed. Keeping levels of vitamin D in prepared foods low enough to make them safe for everybody to consume means that the amount is so minimal it may not be very useful. Research consistently shows that unless vitamin D supplementation is at high enough levels, health improvement doesn't necessarily follow. Low amounts of vitamin D, whether from sunlight, foods, or supplements, may never increase the blood levels to optimal amounts needed by the body.

To make their dietary guidelines seem attainable, the NIH sets the required amount of vitamin D intake pretty low. It advises an adequate intake for all ages from birth to age fifty at 200 IU; for ages fifty-one to seventy at 400 IU; and for those over seventy at 600 IU. The 200 IU level is equal to half a teaspoon of cod liver oil; for the elderly that would equal a teaspoon and a half per day. Aside from cod liver oil, though, how much food, and from what sources, could an eighty-year-old person consume? If not taking a vitamin D supplement, that could mean forty-eight ounces of milk a day, which is probably much more than most elderly people consume.

THE ROLE OF FATS

Relying on food sources of vitamin D—which are often fortified, as in the case of milk—has been our only recourse, but that has been clouded by admonitions against eating fats. Vitamin D is a fat-soluble vitamin, thus it dissolves in fats but not in water. It must have some fat cells for absorption. People with problems absorbing dietary fats won't be able to get much D from sun or supplements. Symptoms of inability to absorb fat include diarrhea and oily stools and can result from several conditions: pancreatic enzyme deficiency; Crohn's disease; cystic fibrosis; celiac disease; liver diseases; and surgical removal of parts of the stomach or intestines. But many more people are unable to absorb fat-soluble vitamins because they are following dietary advice from experts and government health officials (bolstered by advertisers) to eat a low-fat diet. Consuming a low-fat diet or a diet of trans fats (partially hydrogenated plant oils, such as shortening or margarine), without eating the sorts of fats that vitamins A, D, E, K, and other essential nutrients needed for absorption can create a deficiency of fat-soluble vitamins.

Nutritionist and biochemist Mary Enig, author of *Know Your Fats*, explains that one important role of fats in the body is to transport fat-soluble vitamins (A, D, E, and K) and fat-soluble phytochemicals (such as carotenoids—plant pigments that act as antioxidants). She points out that "a low-fat diet can very easily become a vitamin-deficient diet, in part because these vitamins are only found in the fatty (or oily) part of food." Naturally occurring vitamin D is most often found naturally in foods of animal fat origin, such as milk, egg yolk, and pork fat—from animals pastured on green grass. Animals reared indoors in industrial agricultural settings have only minimal amounts of vitamin D received in their feed supplements because they never go into natural sunlight. Vitamin D also appears naturally in fish livers and fatty fish.[33]

Consuming less fat has been the mantra for good health for so long that people are afraid of all fats and are only now recognizing that there's a big difference between "good" fats and "bad" fats. The body needs well-balanced foods that contain essential fatty acids, as well as a proper balance between omega-3 (alpha-linolenic) and omega-6 (linoleic) fatty acids. Omega-6 sources include vegetable seed oils (corn, safflower, soybean); omega-3 sources include flaxseed oil, fish oil, walnuts, and canola oil. These healthy fats, including moderate amounts of meat and dairy products, are healthy fats that help the body retain and utilize the vitamin D absorbed by the sun or in supplements. Trans fats, or hydrogenated fats, in products like margarine and shortening, are now understood as harmful and to be avoided. But quality healthy fats and oils, such as butter and olive oil, remain essential. The book *Fat: It's Not What You Think* by Connie Leas is an excellent source of information about the role healthy fats play in our diet.[34]

Eating a low-fat diet can limit the body's absorption of fat-soluble vitamins, thereby leading to unsatisfactory levels of vitamins A, D, E, and essential fatty acids. One study of five-hundred children found those who ate low-fat diets (diets in which fats made up less than 30 percent of daily intake) were at risk for deficiencies in fat-soluble vitamins. Another study of men eating low-fat (10 percent of intake) vegan diets along with fortified soy protein found they were inadequate in vitamin D levels. In animal studies comparing high-fat versus low-fat diets, those participants who were fed more fats (in the form of vegetable oil) had calcitriol (the active form of vitamin D) levels nearly twice as high as those placed on the low-fat regimen.[35]

For many people, dieting to remain slim and youthful as they age ends up harming their skeleton and other organ functions because they aren't getting adequate quality fat intake. Without quality fats, even supplements won't be utilized in the body as they could be, especially because our digestive system becomes progressively less efficient as we grow older. It's no surprise that falls due to muscle weakness and bone fractures due to brittle, weak bones are a major health problem for older women. When tested, 50 percent of women hospitalized for hip fractures were found to be deficient in vitamin D. One study found that elderly women given vitamin D supplements had a reduced incidence of hip fractures after a two-year period of use. While many authorities recommend low-fat diets for elderly people, the importance of eating high-quality fats and oils is essential to maintaining vitamin D levels as we age.

FATS AND HORMONES

Connie Leas explains why fat cells in the body are so important. Beyond providing energy and building cellular structures, fat cells work as a hormone-producing organ, as part of the endocrine system. Working like the pituitary and the thyroid, fat cells in the body release hormones that affect metabolism, health, and the immune system.[36]

Eating low-fat diets not only hasn't protected us against chronic disease conditions such as heart disease, it has also created a host of other problems because our bodies need to maintain fat cells and the nutrients they store, as well as consume healthy fats. Restricting all fats in the diet in order to lower blood cholesterol levels is no longer linked to preventing heart disease, because the body needs essential healthy fats to function properly.[37]

Dieting to maintain a thin physique image while consuming very little natural healthy fat also wreaks havoc on the body's hormonal and immune systems. Consequently, a bevy of pharmaceuticals have emerged to replace what our body no longer produces naturally.

Hormone replacement therapy (HRT) was once considered a godsend because it appeared to slow down the process of bone deterioration for postmenopausal women. However, significant health risks linked to ovarian cancer brought on by HRT caused the American College of Obstetricians and Gynecologists, the North American Menopause Society, and the American Society for Bone and Mineral Research to recommend that postmenopausal women find some other means of protecting themselves from bone loss. Vitamin D and calcium supplements appear to be safer than HRT.[38]

BACK IN THE SUN

Food sources of vitamin D are elusive, and relying on cholecalciferol supplements is complicated by the fact that we don't really have solid figures for how much vitamin D one should take daily. Sunlight is the solution, but authorities have declared sunlight a carcinogen and warn us to avoid it or don sunglasses, chemical sunscreens, and hats if we choose to venture out. We know how important sunlight is for health, yet how are we to obtain enough natural sunlight, particularly if we live in northern cities or in cloudy areas? Latitude and clouds or pollution—even humidity—can shade us from the full sunlight we need. For example, sunlight exposure from November through February in Boston is insufficient to provide enough vitamin D synthesis in the skin—no matter how many hours of exposure or how little clothing one wears. Anytime there is complete cloud cover, the energy of UV rays is cut in half, and shade reduces it by 60 percent. Sunscreen with a sun protective factor (SPF) of 8 or higher blocks the skin's ability to synthesize vitamin D from sunlight. Industrial pollution also decreases sunlight exposure and may contribute to rickets in children who don't take a vitamin D supplement.

The National Institutes of Health (NIH) advises that individuals can maintain sufficient levels of vitamin D with between five to thirty minutes of sun exposure to the face, arms, legs, or back between 10 AM and 3 PM at least twice a week. Even the NIH advises that "moderate use of commercial tanning beds that emit 2–6% UVB radiation is also effective." If that's not possible, they suggest vitamin D from dietary sources or supplements. The NIH ignores variables such as skin pigmentation, age, or other variables, simplistically advising individuals with limited sun exposure to "include good sources of vitamin D in their diet."[39]

Sunlight remains essential, and researchers are challenging dermatologists who have come down strongly against any sun exposure at all, especially for children and the elderly. Of course getting a sunburn is bad—it destroys skin cells and no one should get burned if it can be prevented. But why do we burn? The key is in our current diet of processed foods and again, the low-fat nutritional campaign waged by various groups to practically rid us of dietary fat altogether.

Many nutritionists advocate consuming more healthy oils and fats to bolster the strength of our cellular walls and to promote skin health. In 1995, a study in Britain provided solid evidence that consuming dietary fish oil rich in omega-3 polyunsaturated fatty acids reduced skin sunburn significantly. Fish oil was also found to be photoprotective, meaning it protected people who were "allergic" to the sun (blisters form on the skin when exposed to sunlight). Fish oils rich in omega-3 also prevented ultraviolet light-induced skin cancer in mice. In the study, people consumed omega-3 fish oils for six months with skin exposure measurements taken before and after beginning the oil regimen. Measured exposure to ultraviolet light showed that these test subjects were significantly less likely to sunburn after consuming the omega-3 fish oil. Participants consumed five capsules (1 gram each) twice daily of oil rich in the eicosapentaenoic and docosahexaenoic acids naturally found in oily fish such as sardines and herring. Omega-3 acts as a buffer to oxidation and cell corrosion by absorbing damage by free radicals and allowing other cellular structures to escape from the negative impact of free radical damage. Their ability to inhibit free radicals could explain why omega-3s work as anti-inflammatory agents in rheumatoid arthritis, as well. Animal studies have shown omega-3 from fish oil to inhibit UV-induced skin cancers in animals.[40]

Diet may be the crucial element in restoring skin health so that we can safely make our own vitamin D by exposing ourselves to full sunlight. Long-term studies on the effect of omega-3 fatty acids in preventing skin cancer in humans are crucial. Slathering ourselves in chemical sunscreen to prevent sunburn, thereby reducing the incidence of skin cancer, only ignores the biological causes for our increased susceptibility to both. Sunscreen and sun avoidance are patchwork solutions that ignore the physiological cause—lack of omega-3 food sources—that developed as we changed our cultural dietary patterns. Only Japanese and Norwegian diets currently provide adequate amounts of fish intake to maintain adequate vitamin D levels during winter. For the rest of us, replacing traditional oily fish meals (cod, salmon, sardines) with burgers, pasta, and pizza means we're unable to maintain the health our ancestors did through diet alone.[41]

SKIN PIGMENTATION

Skin, like other organs, isn't static. We're continually replacing dead cells with new ones in a process that takes between two to four weeks to replace the entire epidermal (surface layer) of one's skin. Melanin, the pigment that gives skin its particular color, is produced by epidermal cells for an important reason: it absorbs ultraviolet rays. Melanin, which gives skin its tan or brown tone, is a protective device that allows individuals who have enough of it to spend long periods in direct sunlight without burning. Melanin forms a protective veil over the body, facing outward on the skin's surface, shielding the cellular DNA from ultraviolet light. In some people melanin forms in patches, creating freckles, and as we age it appears as patches of spots (sometimes referred to as liver or age spots), particularly on hands and forearms. Everyone has some melanin pigment except people with albinism, the absence of melanin in skin, hair, and eyes.[42]

People with less melanin, or lighter skin coloring, are more susceptible to skin cancers than those with darker pigment. People with lighter skin coloring need less time in the sun to develop adequate D levels, while those with darker skins need more time in sunlight for optimal health. Pale skin will reach optimal vitamin D levels in twenty minutes of full sun exposure. After that, the skin resists making more D and may simply burn instead. It takes three to six times longer for dark skin to reach the same saturation level. Despite the fact that the amount of D one gets from sunlight exposure varies depending upon season, time of day, and a host of other variables, the need for darker-pigmented people to attain longer exposures is clear. Particularly, dark-skinned African Americans need to get much more sunlight than most do; and if they live in the cloudy northern regions, it's practically impossible for them to get adequate sunlight exposure. African American men and women in the United States have significantly lower vitamin D levels than whites due to the high melanin content of their skin that filters UV rays, and because they don't consume as much vitamin D in fortified foods (like milk and cold cereal) or through supplements. Mexican Americans have similar low levels of vitamin D and lower vitamin D intakes from diet or supplements.

Higher than average rates of certain cancers, hypertension, and other chronic conditions experienced by African Americans and dark-skinned individuals living in northern latitudes can very likely be directly linked to their inadequate D levels. Rickets is appearing among dark-pigmented infants, particularly those who have been breastfed and who don't receive vitamin D supplements. In the early twentieth century, rickets was almost universal among African American infants living in the northern United States, and while it receded with food fortification, there's been a resurgence of rickets among breastfed infants in the north and dark-skinned infants anywhere in the country. A recent study in Columbus Hill, a black community in New York City, found that most black breastfed infants not given cod liver oil supplements developed rickets.[43]

PIGMENT, HEALTH, AND VITAMIN D

Mortality rates for prostate cancer are markedly higher among black men than white; in fact, American males with West/Central African ancestry have the highest prostate cancer rate in the world, and at a younger age than other males. Yet, in West Africa, males have among the world's lowest rates of prostate cancer. In 1990, researchers first proposed that prostate cancer was caused by vitamin D deficiency; recent findings support that idea. It appears that the ability of vitamin D to control cell changes and the rate of cell growth directly affects the incidence of prostate cancer. Just as with rickets, the geographic and ecologic link to prostate disease was identified before experimental research could validate it.

The issue of healthcare and racism is a highly controversial topic. African American health problems are exacerbated by availability and quality of healthcare, but the issue is even broader. By ignoring race in healthcare, biological differences due to skin melanin content, and the need that dark-skinned individuals have for increased vitamin D supplementation at northern latitudes, healthcare systems fail dark-skinned individuals. Kathleen Fuller, a medical anthropologist in Arizona, tackled the issue of healthcare and racism recently, pointing out that "reframing the problem of health disparities from one of race and racism to one of phenotype/environmental mismatch permits a solution to an otherwise intractable problem." Lumping together individuals into a culturally constructed "race" means that it's difficult to create vitamin D guidelines to suit diverse groups of people. Because the range of skin pigmentation among African Americans is extremely wide, their vitamin D needs can be quite different.

For people with dark-pigmented skin, living at northern latitudes without taking vitamin D supplements can spell havoc for health and can even be deadly. Hypertension, prostate cancer, breast cancer, multiple sclerosis, low–birth weight infants, cesarean childbirth, and rickets are all disorders related to inadequate sunlight or vitamin D, and all occur more frequently among people with darker pigmentation. Even dark-skinned children in Jamaica developed rickets because their lifestyle prevented them from getting adequate outdoor sunlight exposure or consuming sufficient amounts of fortified foods.[44]

The high incidence of low–birth weight black infants has long puzzled health authorities because it crossed socioeconomic lines. It's been recently linked to hypertension, a condition twice as common among American women with West/Central African ancestry as women of European ancestry. Also, a low level of vitamin D in the mother's body has been identified as a factor in slow fetus growth, because it limits the amount of calcium passed from mother to child through the placenta, leading to low–birth weight infants.

Fuller suggests a new way to view health and race—one in which individual biology and residential environment take precedence. She points out that dark pigmentation creates similar healthcare dynamics for South Asians, Central/West Africans, and native Australians, yet none are culturally linked via race. Rather than create culturally defined racial categories for healthcare, she suggests basing medical decisions on pigmentation, something that can be easily monitored with a spectrophotometer (which measures light intensity and wavelength) and computer in about three seconds, and can be easily added to a patient's medical records. Using pigmentation levels as a substitute for racial designation on healthcare forms would allow more accurate treatment. Heavily pigmented individuals living in Seattle would have more in common, health wise, than a group of lightly pigmented individuals in the same location, and their health needs could be addressed more precisely. Pigmentation levels can be as important as blood typing in developing treatment and prevention plans. As Fuller points out, "Hypertension could then be addressed in an appropriate biological manner, rather than an inappropriate racial one." And we could eliminate such inequities as the federal government's mandate that everyone should avoid more than fifteen minutes of sun exposure per day, a guideline that may work for pale-skinned individuals but ignores the need of dark-skinned people for three times as much exposure in order to be healthy.[45]

VITAMIN D AND RACIAL DIFFERENCES

RACIAL DIFFERENCES IN VITAMIN D CHART

Racial differences in vitamin D status, intakes, food sources, and supplement use in white and black adults in the United States; results from the third National Health and Nutrition Examination Survey, 1988–1994.[46]

	White adults	Black adults
Sample size	6456	4316
Vitamin D level in blood test	25(OH)D79 nmol/L	48.2 nmol/L
Vitamin D intake from supplements alone	2.84 microgram/d	2.00 microgram/d
Vitamin D intake from food and supplements (fortified milk and cereals)	7.92 microgram/d	6.20 microgram/d
Vitamin D intake from milk	1.86 microgram/d	.92 microgram/d

The current Daily Recommended Intake of vitamin D is 5 micrograms (200 IU).

SKIN CANCERS

This new vitamin D research will help the medical profession and the public to recognize that sunlight is not the deadly agent they once thought; that indoor lifestyles brought about by long working hours, home media, and lack of outdoor parks and facilities are the problem, exacerbated by our diet, which lacks vitamin D sources, as well as adequate minerals and essential fats. Yet the problem of sun-related skin cancer makes us hesitate to sun ourselves, no matter how much we need it.

The government entity that oversees nutrition and health is the Food and Drug Administration, and the FDA is adamantly against anyone basking in sunlight. FDA spokespersons work closely with the American Academy of Dermatologists to warn against sunlight exposure or using ultraviolet tanning beds and sunlamps. Public health officials warn people to avoid going out in the sun between the hours of 10 AM and 4 PM; to wear hats, long pants, and long-sleeved shirts; to use sunglasses with 100 percent UV protection; and to wear a sunscreen with an SPF of 15 or higher. They also warn people to get the ultraviolet index for their location from the daily newspaper to better avoid going out on sunny days.

Why the concern with sunlight exposure when it's so necessary for health and well-being? Skin cancer is the only issue, and yet in spite of repeated mantras about sun exposure causing skin cancer, it has not been completely proven. Skin cancer appears in two general types: malignant melanoma (which spreads to other parts of the body, usually the lymph nodes and liver, and has a high mortality rate) and nonmelanoma (appearing as either basal cell carcinoma or squamous cell carcinoma). Melanoma, the more dangerous of the three, usually shows up on skin areas that never were exposed to the sun, such as thighs, abdomen, even inside the eye or on the soles of the feet. Melanoma appears more often in people who never go into the sun than those who do. The other kinds of skin cancer, the carcinomas, are found mostly in fair-skinned people of northern European-Celtic ancestry, appearing on the nose and top of the ears. While carcinomas are ugly and sometimes painful, that type of cancer is seldom life-threatening and can be removed surgically. It is related to overexposure to sunlight by skin that burns easily. Wearing a hat can prevent it.

The relationship between sunlight and skin cancer is puzzling. The number of skin cancer cases began accelerating in the 1970s for reasons no one has been able to explain. Some researchers speculated that it was due to the invention of the bikini, but that hardly seems like a societal shift. In fact, people are not going into the sun more; rather, they're staying indoors for even greater amounts of the time, due to indoor malls, shopping centers, indoor pools and exercise centers, and even indoor playgrounds for children. So as the numbers of melanoma cases increase, the number of people going outdoors for any amount of time has declined.

Meanwhile, the facts favor more sunlight exposure rather than less if we are to fight many types of cancer. General cancer rates are much higher at higher latitudes than in places closer to the equator, and the cancers connected to vitamin D deficiency are more deadly. Cancers linked to low D levels—breast, colon, and prostate—claim many times more. It's a delicate trade-off, but the cancer numbers suggest getting more sunlight is a benefit. You can see the following chart showing the number of deaths annually from cancers linked to low vitamin D levels compared to skin cancer deaths.

CANCER DEATH RATES (2004)

Type of Cancer	Deaths
Skin cancer (melanoma)	7, 952
Ovarian cancer	14,716
Prostate cancer	29,002
Breast cancer	40,954
Colon cancer	44,988

Source: US Cancer Statistics, National Vital Statistics Reports, Center for Disease Control.

There are about a million estimated new cases of skin cancer each year in the United States, of which 80 percent are basal cell type, the one least likely to be fatal. The American Academy of Dermatology estimates about 7,200 deaths per year are due to malignant melanoma, the most fatal type of skin cancer. During the past fifty years, incidents of both types have increased significantly in the United States, Britain, and Australia—countries where light-skinned Caucasians make up the majority of the population. Pale-skinned people are at greater risk for sunburn and sun-related aging of the skin, and for years all three countries have engaged in federally supported programs to warn against sun exposure and sunburn. Australia's "SunSmart" campaign has been ongoing for twenty-five years. The public health programs have been based on the belief that reducing a person's cumulative exposure to direct sunlight will reduce the likelihood of developing skin cancer.[47]

The sun-avoidance message, however, has its critics. Dermatologists concerned with skin health strongly support the message to avoid sun exposure, while endocrinologists and nutritionists argue for the benefits of sun exposure to the rest of the body. More research is emerging every month through the major medical journals to support the idea that vitamin D—from sunshine—plays a valuable role in preventing cancer, including skin cancer.

New research on sun exposure turns the sun-avoidance dogma on its head. The greatest risk factor for malignant melanoma is the presence of many large, abnormal moles, which change shape and color. Moles have no relationship to sunlight exposure. Several studies have found that in some way, sunlight and vitamin D appear to mediate the development of melanomas.[48] A Connecticut-based study of more than five hundred melanoma patients over a five-year period found that those with the most sun exposure—even severe sunburns or high levels of intermittent sun exposure—were *less* likely to die from melanoma than individuals who had never been severely sunburned or who had low levels of intermittent sun exposure. Sun exposure and survival from melanoma seem connected to vitamin D and its actions to block the multiplication of cells and slow down cell death; vitamin D increases one's survival chances from melanoma. Sunlight's effect against melanoma appears to be similar to the relationship between low vitamin D levels and mortality from cancers such as prostate, breast, colon, and ovary. Australian researchers suggest strong associations between non-Hodgkin lymphoma and sun exposure, hypothesizing that sunlight creates vitamin D as a protective mechanism against that disease. Australian researchers found that vitamin D actually protects the DNA in human skin cells from UV radiation damage.[49]

SUNLIGHT PREVENTS CANCER

Sun exposure to prevent cancer is nothing new; it was first suggested in the 1930s and 1940s, when rates of skin and internal cancers were found to be inversely related to sun exposure. In the early 1990s, epidemiological studies showed breast and prostate cancer death rates were linked to distance from the equator. Today, we're finally getting the laboratory findings to prove sunlight and vitamin D's activity as a chemopreventive agent, spurring the development of synthetic analogs that can be directed precisely at certain cancers.[50]

We're also discovering that skin tanning has a function in preventing the development of skin cancer. Researchers at Dana-Farber Cancer Institute found that the protein p53, which plays a role in causing the skin to tan after sun exposure, also reduces the risk of melanoma. The ability to tan seems to be a protective factor against skin cancer. "The number one risk factor for melanoma is an inability to tan," said Dr. David E. Fisher, director of the Melanoma Program at Dana-Farber. The study showed that p53, which is a tumor-suppressor protein in the skin, "has a powerful role in protecting us against sun damage in the skin," according to Fisher. In a complex reaction within the skin cells, p53 levels in the cells rise after skin exposure to sunlight, sparking a process within the skin that triggers secretion of a hormone that causes melanin to change skin color, creating a tan. The tanning process is only one aspect of p53's activity after sunlight exposure, however. Somehow it also triggers a rise in the production of endorphins, which create feelings of pleasure. This activity, still not fully understood, may explain why people feel good after a session of sunning and why people unconsciously seek out sunlight exposure.[51]

Accepting the idea we need plenty of sunshine for health is one part of the solution; how to obtain it is another. If we simply can't get enough vitamin D from scanty sunlight in fall and winter, how do we remain naturally healthy? Tests in Europe showed that children and young adults, those most likely to be outdoors, have insufficient D levels in winter; elderly and institutionalized people experience insufficient D levels throughout the year; and people living in northern cities, such as Boston and Seattle, have few days (year-round) with adequate levels of UV penetration, even if they spent all their time outdoors. With inadequate levels of D linked to osteoporosis, tuberculosis, rheumatoid arthritis, multiple sclerosis, inflammatory bowel diseases, high blood pressure, as well as specific cancers, perhaps the FDA and dermatologists should rethink their position. As a preventive, D reduces blood pressure, improves blood glucose in diabetes, and shows improvement in multiple sclerosis and rheumatoid arthritis.[52]

We're still on the frontiers of understanding how ultraviolet radiation affects the body and how to manipulate or turn it into a commercial substance in order to control the benefits. At this point, we're not much farther along than we were in the 1930s, when light therapy, food fortification, and supplements made by irradiation became the mainstays of vitamin D treatment.

So, for most of the year, people in northern latitudes should get as much sun exposure as possible, without sunscreen, and if worried about aging their skin, wear a hat to cover their face while exposing their legs. Indeed, no one should allow themselves to be burned by the sun. Sun exposure requires healthy skin, however, so strengthening skin cells by consuming more omega-3 essential fatty acids, eating healthy amounts of quality fats and oils (such as butter, olive and nut oil, eggs, whole milk) so vitamin D metabolizes and stores well in the body, and taking vitamin D supplements in amounts consistent with personal vitamin D requirements is a sensible solution. Our relationship to sunlight depends upon our age, skin color, geographic location, and lifestyle pattern. No "one-size-fits-all" will work for everyone.[53]

Chapter Five

A PANDORA'S BOX OF AILMENTS

I n the past, vitamin D deficiency brought to mind weak bones and unfortunate children with rickets, so public health efforts were directed to get kids drinking fortified milk—and parents to supply them with it. It seemed to be a problem limited to parents and maybe school lunch directors. But current research on vitamin D has exploded the old idea that children are the only ones who need vitamin D. A recent international symposium on vitamin D was titled "Bone and Beyond," highlighting the new recognition that vitamin D is essential to many tissues, organs, and body processes other than bone health.[1]

While vitamin D is known to be necessary to balance minerals for bone and muscle use—what might be called the "classic" vitamin D role—the new information about vitamin D's action throughout the body has led researchers to implicate its depletion in several chronic disease conditions ranging from nervous system disorders to heart disease, obesity, high blood pressure, multiple sclerosis, diabetes, and cancer. Going beyond sunlight's classic effects on osteoporosis and rickets, this chapter will examine the various chronic disease conditions and their relationship to low vitamin D levels.

A NEW EPIDEMIC

Along with discovering how important vitamin D is throughout the body, new research points to what some are calling an epidemic of vitamin D deficiency.[2] Rickets, long believed lost to history, has emerged again. The first cases recognized occurred in the American South: six cases appeared in Georgia between 1997 and 1999, and another thirty in North Carolina between 1998 and 1999. Other studies echoed the findings, revealing that rickets had indeed returned and was no longer a disease of the poor. Suburban children, particularly babies with darker-pigmented skin who were breastfed without vitamin D supplementation or children of mothers with vitamin D deficiency, all living in far northern (or in the case of Argentina and South Africa, in the far southern regions) were developing symptoms of rickets.[3]

Along with rickets, osteoporosis and a host of other problems have developed because people aren't consuming enough calcium, getting enough sunlight, or supplementing with vitamin D. According to Michael Holick, a leading vitamin D researcher at the Boston University School of Medicine, "A minimum of 25 percent of adolescents and adults in this country are vitamin D deficient." A University of Maine study found almost 50 percent of teenage girls were deficient in vitamin D during winter months and 17 percent were deficient during the sunny months of summer. Among healthy adults in Calgary, Canada, 34 percent tested positive for vitamin D deficiency. Other studies found that 45 percent of Australian nursing home residents were deficient in vitamin D. Asians living in the United Kingdom had blood levels tested to reveal that 85 percent were deficient in winter months, and 38 percent were still deficient even in summer. Pakistani women living in Norway were tested and 83 percent were deficient.[4]

In 2003, the National Institutes of Health (NIH) sponsored a major conference, pulling together experts from wide-ranging health fields who looked at the many gaps in knowledge about vitamin D and laid out research agendas for the future to identify how much vitamin D the body needs, establish accurate measurements, and revise recommended daily levels of vitamin D. The research base is solid and significant; the problem ahead is how to overcome what the conference termed the "public information shortfall," because consumers receive conflicting advice from experts regarding sun exposure, taking vitamin supplements, and breastfeeding without vitamin D supplementation.[5]

In 2004, a group of experimental biologists convened to address vitamin D insufficiency and chronic diseases, adding to the number of researchers asking for new definitions of vitamin D adequacy. What brought the issue home to the medical community, however, was a study done on physicians working in Portland, Oregon, hospitals. Medical residents, a group considered most likely among the population to be healthy, had low vitamin D levels—at least half had vitamin D levels considered inadequate (they tested at less than 20 ng/mL on the calcidiol test).[6] Physicians are as vulnerable to low vitamin D levels as the rest of us because of long working hours and lack of sunlight exposure.

Without taking adequate supplements, they were setting themselves up for long-term health problems.

The Portland study alerted medical professionals to their own vulnerability to sunlight deficiency while other more recent findings dispel longtime views about who is at risk for vitamin D deficiency. It is no longer considered a problem limited to women and children. An Arizona study found that not only do men suffer from osteoporosis, just as women do, but that the rate of bone fracture over age fifty was actually slightly higher for men than women. Bone strength and health, the classic measure of vitamin D activity in the body, has become a huge problem as the United States population ages.[7]

DEFICIENCY IN SUNNY CLIMATES

The availability of sunlight is a drawback: in Britain and Scandinavia, as in other northern latitudes, there simply isn't enough of the right type of sunlight during winter to make adequate vitamin D in the skin (even with exposure to sunlight). In northern latitude cities such as Minneapolis or Montreal, little vitamin D can be created naturally from sunshine between October and the end of March. Even people living in sunny climates often suffer vitamin D deficiency, though, simply because they do not go out into the sunlight or live where a haze of pollution deflects UV rays.

For example, in Delhi, India, excessive numbers of healthy people were found to have low vitamin D levels, even while living in a sunny climate. Vitamin D deficiency is prevalent in India, which is surprising because it's a tropical country with abundant sunshine. In Saudi Arabia, a land of intense sunshine, studies find people have low vitamin D levels because they avoid sunlight exposure, remaining indoors or wearing protective clothing much of the time. India requires no vitamin D supplementation in processed foods; Saudi Arabia requires vitamin D be added to margarine.[8]

CALCIUM CONNECTION

Admittedly, not all cases of rickets are due to lack of sunlight. Calcium, phosphorus, and magnesium combine with vitamin D to create a necessary nutritional balance. For example, Nigerian children and others in the African Sahel are experiencing increasing numbers of rickets cases, which in this instance isn't related to a lack of vitamin D (they have plenty of sunlight), but instead the condition is due to insufficient levels of dietary calcium. As they shift away from a traditional cattle-based diet to cheaper grains, the Nigerians have few significant sources of calcium in their diet. In sunny Istanbul, too, children suffer rickets because they lack both calcium and vitamin D. Clearly, in many urban settings, children aren't going outdoors enough to get vitamin D and their diet provides little calcium. High-rise urban slums and crowded shanty-towns, even in the sunniest of cities, provide no opportunities for children to enjoy sunshine at playgrounds or parks.[9]

Some groups have adapted genetically to their traditional diet and latitude, requiring less calcium than believed essential for well-being, according to widely accepted calcium intake levels. The Alaskan Inuit, the Chinese, and the Thai peoples have a different adaptation to calcium, which allows them to absorb more calcium intestinally than do other groups of people. Children eating traditional diets in these cultures ingest significantly less calcium than their counterparts in the United States, but because they have a genetic adaptation that utilizes calcium more efficiently, their bones are strong and healthy. As the Inuit children in one study began adopting a "market" diet, consuming higher levels of calcium daily, they actually became ill. Higher levels of hypercalcuria (abnormally high levels of calcium excreted in the urine) and kidney problems resulted from consuming levels of calcium recommended for average consumption by the general North American population. Several servings of milk daily, or calcium supplements, actually can be detrimental to those with a genetic adaptation to traditionally low consumption of calcium. Along with calcium, their bodies seem programmed to get along well with lower amounts of sunlight, too. The number of vitamin D receptor genotypes (found in Inuit children and similarly in some Asian populations) is much lower than the average Caucasian population. That means their cells have fewer receptors that react to the vitamin D in the bloodstream. Fewer receptors mean they must function more efficiently to get the same cellular work done. It appears that the specific gene, known as *bb*, allows for more efficient absorption of calcium in the intestine. So Inuit children and others with similar inherited cell makeup can only absorb as much vitamin D as their cells allow, which is the correct amount for survival in their particular traditional environment.[10]

In the modern era, people shifted away from local foods to eat a diet of foods grown and processed elsewhere, but their bodies didn't easily make the switch. Margarine, canned food, and refined sugar are examples of foods containing few minerals and poor fats, which leave their mark in stature, weight gain, tooth decay, and vision problems, among other effects.

As adults and children around the globe drink an increasing amount of sugared soft drinks, they consume less milk. As they adopt refined wheat flour in baked goods and noodles, they shift away from traditional foods, particularly fish, organ meats (such as tripe and kidneys), and vegetables. For children whose bones are forming, it's a potential disaster. For adults, it means decades of declining health. Corn-sweetened soda, juice-flavored drinks, and margarine have eliminated calcium from many diets, while television and indoor work keep people out of sunlight, even in areas that receive high amounts of sunlight year-round.

TOOTH DECAY

Vitamin D deficiency is an elusive condition to identify because it affects so many body processes and can take years to become evident, often being mistaken for other health problems. One of the clearest indicators of vitamin D deficiency appears in our teeth. While the same damage is going on inside the body, our teeth are completely visible, so their condition can provide a window into the body's interior. In the 1920s, May Mellanby, who worked with dogs in the first experiments to recognize the relationship between rickets and sunlight, linked tooth decay to lack of sunlight and found it was exacerbated by a diet that included large amounts of grain, particularly oatmeal. After examining two thousand sections of teeth from 1,400 dogs, she published photographs of dogs' mouths showing decay, lack of enamel, crumbling teeth, and malformed dentition. She turned to examining children's baby teeth, obtaining over a thousand from dentists and realized that more than two-thirds were severely undeveloped, with 85 percent showing decay. She studied children in a London tuberculosis hospital, adding cereal to the diets of some and cod liver oil, irradiated ergosterol (vitamin D_2), milk, and egg yolk to others. Tooth decay halted and teeth hardened in proportion to the amount of vitamin D added to the children's diets.

Weston Price, the itinerant dentist-turned-anthropologist, gauged dietary inadequacies by looking at people's teeth. He traveled to remote areas of the world, examining people's teeth to prove his hypothesis that a modern diet of commercially processed foods was causing tooth decay. Price found rampant decay, malformed teeth and mouths, and a general change in facial structure between generations with adequate D levels and others without it.

He also realized that while people's diets varied depending upon where they lived, their indigenous diets provided them with four times the amount of minerals and water-soluble vitamins (C and B-complex) as the standard American diet of the 1930s. More astounding, he found traditional diets contained ten times the amount of fat-soluble vitamins (such as vitamins D, A, and K) found in the animal fats Americans ate. Traditional diets that included butterfat from cows grazing in green grass, fish liver oils, fish eggs (often dried in the sun), and organ meats (including liver, kidney, and parts of the digestive tract) provided the older generation with a healthful edge, including strong, well-formed teeth. When the next generation switched to eating canned foods, flour, sugar, hydrogenated oils and margarines, and skim milk, their teeth reflected the change immediately with increased cavities, inadequate jaw development, and eventual tooth loss.[11]

Today, it's not at all unusual for preschoolers to have several cavities filled in their primary teeth before their adult teeth even appear. Good dental care means getting fillings or caps applied to children's decaying teeth. Brushing, flossing, and fluoride in toothpaste have become standard dental hygiene, taught in schools and reinforced during annual dental checkups. Yet parents aren't always told how important calcium, vitamin D, and sunlight are to tooth formation. Strong teeth don't happen from the outside-in. Rather, the building process starts deep inside the tooth, where cells lay down solid structure for a tooth that's resistant to decay and wear. Enamel on the outside protects the tooth from changes in saliva acidity as well as grinding and chipping injuries. Worn teeth, weak enamel, and teeth that fracture easily are signs of a mineral and vitamin D insufficiency. It's a structural problem, and adding fluoride to public drinking water or toothpaste won't solve it.[12]

In the 1930s, studies done comparing children's dental health in school classrooms lit with full-spectrum lightbulbs (which are similar to natural sunlight) showed a decline in tooth decay compared to regular classrooms with incandescent or fluorescent lighting. At the end of the school year, the children in classrooms illuminated by full-spectrum bulbs had fewer cavities than their counterparts in the other classrooms. All the children were drinking from a public water supply fortified with fluoride. In the 1950s, classroom studies showed similar results.[13]

Tooth decay in children was also found to have a seasonal connection, with the incidence of cavities sharply higher in the winter-spring period than in the summer-fall, when children's vitamin D stores are naturally highest from sunlight exposure. Researchers discovered that a simple vitamin D supplement could alleviate tooth decay. When children were given varying amounts of vitamin D in the diet, there was a proportional decrease in the number of cavities. Children were given vitamin D supplements in amounts of 200 IU, 400 IU, and 800 IU per day, with results showing that 200 IU was not enough in keeping tooth decay down to summer levels. Supplementing with 800 IU per day was necessary to offset the lack of sunlight during the winter-spring months, keeping tooth decay levels down during the darkest months of the year. Those amounts are significantly higher than the government's recommended daily allowance (RDA) for a child, which currently is set at 200 IU daily for everyone under age fifty. The connection between sunlight (or vitamin D supplements) and strong teeth was made over half a century ago—in the 1930s—yet today it's virtually ignored.[14]

THE SKELETAL-MUSCULAR SYSTEM AND VITAMIN D

Osteomalacia was recognized in the early twentieth century as a condition in adults that was caused by the same factors as rickets in children. Osteomalacia is softening of the bones caused by insufficient levels of vitamin D or by problems with the body's ability to absorb and use vitamin D. The softer bones have normal amounts of collagen, which gives the bones their structure, but they lack the minerals that give bones their strength. While lack of vitamin D affects growing children, causing a variety of health effects such as limited growth, misshaped bones, decaying teeth, and more, it also causes problems for adults, but since adults have stopped growing longer bones and new teeth, the condition exhibits different effects and is termed osteomalacia. Adult bones are no longer growing but are always undergoing remodeling, meaning that bone tissue is continuously being replaced by new bone, a process that requires a steady supply of calcium, magnesium, and phosphorus, minerals all regulated by vitamin D. When calcium levels in the bloodstream drop too low, parathyroid hormones instruct the bones to release calcium in order to increase blood calcium levels. The calcium goes out to other vital processes (including the circulatory system), while the bones sit like empty piggybanks, waiting for a refill when more calcium is ingested. If that doesn't happen, or if enough vitamin D isn't obtained to regulate the process, calcium isn't replenished and the bones weaken.

When osteomalacia is present the bones soften from lack of vitamin D until they can no longer support standing and walking. It's a progressive decalcification of bony tissues, often causing bone pain. The lack of vitamin D means calcium isn't utilized and the bones eventually soften because the body extracts calcium from the most accessible source, our bones. If left untreated it can become an irreversible condition.

Since our bodies are continually using and replacing calcium, we are always at risk if we do not have adequate amounts of it, along with the vitamin D to use it effectively. Along with a rising number of children afflicted with rickets, adults with bone problems related to vitamin D deficiency are also growing in number. Osteoporosis, the adult bone disorder most people are familiar with, has increased substantially in recent years. As of 2003, there were about 3.6 million people diagnosed with osteoporosis, compared with half a million cases in 1994. That's just the tip of the iceberg, according to the National Osteoporosis Foundation, which estimates that 10 million Americans are afflicted with the condition and face a high risk of bone fractures. Osteoporosis is different from osteomalacia in that it is a loss of bone tissue rather than a softening, resulting in brittle bones that fracture very easily. It's common in elderly individuals and postmenopausal women and results in shorter stature and frail skeletal structure as one ages. It can be caused by a lack of vitamin D and calcium, the inability of the body to assimilate D and calcium from the diet, or from taking steroid medications. It has become a major problem in Western nations as greater numbers of people enter their elder years and of concern to healthcare practitioners because it is often underdiagnosed and undertreated.[15]

DANGEROUS FALLS AND FRACTURES

A large problem for the aging population today is the combination of falls and fractures. Bone fractures in the elderly are due to two risk factors: osteoporosis and the fall itself. Osteoporosis alone doesn't cause broken bones, so the act of falling is a primary concern. Calcium plays a major role in maintaining muscle strength and resiliency, which maintains movement, balance, and coordination. Falls due to weak muscle strength and the resultant fractures due to osteoporosis are both linked to low levels of vitamin D. About 50 percent of people over seventy years of age suffer from inadequate levels of vitamin D, leading to less muscle strength, poor ligament tone, and poor balance—all making people prone to falling. Once they hit the ground, their weakened and brittle bones, due to inadequate mineralization, are more prone to fracture. In this regard, simple falls from a standing position are a public health burden because they create long-term medical consequences. Researchers in Finland point out that while a simple fall isn't as traumatic as a motor vehicle collision, the severity of the outcome is comparable because the force of the fall clearly exceeds the breaking strength of the bone. They suggest calling such fall-related injuries "fall-induced high-impact injuries" rather than minimal-trauma fractures.

Balance training and dietary supplements with vitamin D and calcium have been successful in preventing the initial fall, therefore eliminating the likely bone breaks. Australian researchers gave vitamin D and calcium supplements to nursing home residents for two years and found significant reduction in the number and rate of falls, even for those not considered vitamin D deficient. They recommended 1000 IU of vitamin D and 600 mg of calcium carbonate daily. Taking 400 IU of vitamin D daily, the current recommended standard, was not considered sufficient to prevent fractures from falls.[16]

CHILDREN'S WEAK BONES

Although most degenerative skeletal ailments affect adults, children are experiencing another bone-related health problem besides the resurgence of childhood rickets. The condition is nameless and difficult to pinpoint or diagnose, but youngsters' bones have noticeably weakened, with a corresponding rise in the number of children arriving at emergency rooms with broken bones. A recent study showed that more than 40 percent of doctors encountered an increase in fractures among children and young people under age eighteen. Two other medical studies reveal the rate of broken arms has soared, up by more than 50 percent in girls and 30 percent in boys since 1970. "What used to be bruises are more likely to be breaks nowadays," says Celia Brown, who practices general family medicine in California and teaches at UCLA. "Kids just aren't developing adequate bone mass." The National Institute of Child Health and Human Development (NICHHD) calls it a "calcium crisis" and points to increased intake of milk as a solution.[17]

Culturally, dairy products remain Americans' major source of calcium, but young people aren't drinking milk. Studies show 86 percent of teen girls and 64 percent of teen boys aren't getting enough calcium each day because they are consuming less than the daily recommended equivalent of four glasses of milk. It's a crisis with serious consequences in the near future. Describing the new wave of osteoporosis among youth as "a pediatric disease with geriatric consequences," Duane Alexander, director of the NICHHD, points out that preventing bone problems begins in childhood. He warns that because of poor diets, "today's children and teens are certain to face a serious public health problem in the future." Young people around the world have shifted away from old-fashioned milk drinks to highly advertised status drinks such as sodas, sugared juices, and "sport drinks." The results won't be far off in the future. Alexander warns, "as these children get older, this calcium crisis will become more serious as the population starts to show its highest rate of osteoporosis and other bone health problems in our nation's history."[18]

But it's not inevitable; it's entirely preventable. More calcium, along with sunshine and vitamin D supplements, can save billions of dollars in future health expenses as well as human suffering. Without action, today's youth are slated to be the cohorts of worn and fragile "old people" before they reach middle age.

VITAMIN D AND MUSCLES

How vitamin D works in our muscle tissue is still a mystery. At the molecular level it appears that vitamin D and calcium work together to regulate the proliferation, maturation, and function of muscle through signals to the genes. Muscle weakness responds well to vitamin D and calcium supplements, and new findings show that a high intake of vitamin D can actually improve muscle strength. Not only can "bodybuilders" benefit from vitamin D, it increases muscle volume in the elderly and can be useful for dieters who want more muscle and a better-toned body. Without adequate calcium, regulated by vitamin D, muscles don't function well, becoming weak and atrophied, or brittle and inelastic. When both are in adequate supply, muscles are resilient and strong, maintaining the body's erect posture and flexible mobility. Ample amounts of vitamin D and daily calcium intake of at least 500 mg can help prevent mobility problems that come with aging. If you can't get up quickly from a chair (the timed-up-and-go test, or TUG), pay attention to your vitamin D and calcium levels. Perhaps a blood test for vitamin D is in order.

Bone density declines more quickly during winter than summer, because vitamin D levels drop during that time, but with supplementation at 800 IU/day combined with calcium the decline it can be slowed. Such a regimen will also reduce fracture risk in adults over age sixty-five. Even before bone density starts to improve, supplementing the diet with this level of vitamin D can increase the muscle and ligament tone enough to improve strength and balance, thereby reducing the occurrence of fractures by about a third.[19]

BEYOND BONES: NEUROLOGICAL AND PSYCHOLOGICAL DEVELOPMENT

While it's been easier to recognize the role that the lack of vitamin D plays in bone loss, muscle weakness, and reduced mineral metabolism, exploring its negative effects on brain development, cognition, and mental illness is a new frontier. Inadequate vitamin D levels have been associated with physical decline and are increasingly being linked to mental development, too.[20] It doesn't appear that low vitamin D levels affect cognitive performance in adolescents or adults, meaning learning and memory tasks aren't impaired if one's vitamin D levels are inadequate. But it does look like one's early brain development can be affected by both the mother's level of vitamin D while pregnant as well as the level of vitamin D during childhood.

There is a plethora of rat studies showing clear effects of slowed brain development due to inadequate levels of prenatal vitamin D. Since D controls the number of brain cells that are produced as well as how quickly cells are discarded and replaced, inadequate levels of the vitamins in babies and the very young could have serious repercussions. It's the same activity vitamin D uses to kill cancer cells elsewhere in the body, but in the brain it works to facilitate normal development. The brain structure, cell density, and transmission of chemical nerve impulses were all impaired in rats whose mothers were vitamin D deficient. When those baby rats were later given adequate amounts of vitamin D, they failed to overcome the brain deficits they had demonstrated at birth. It appears that inadequate prenatal vitamin D can disrupt brain development in a manner that cannot be overcome with later intervention.[21] Not only were brain cells modified, but it also appears that when rats born to vitamin D–deficient mothers grew to adulthood, they exhibited hyperlocomotion, or hyperactivity, as well as subtle behavioral changes in learning and memory when tested in laboratory settings.

While no human studies are conclusive at this point, there's a lot of interest in detecting links between vitamin D, brain development, and conditions such as autism and schizophrenia. Both conditions have become increasingly common over the past decades, apparently corresponding to the increasing medical advice to avoid the sun, according to John Cannell, psychiatrist at the Atascadero State Hospital in California. Cannell postulates a link between autism and diminished vitamin D, pointing to the animal data that show severe vitamin D deficiency during gestation creates havoc with proteins involved in brain development, leading to increased brain size and enlarged ventricles, similar to the brains of autistic children. He points out that autism is more frequent in areas where ultraviolet-B rays are blocked, such as higher latitudes, urban areas, and regions covered by pollution or precipitation. Adding support to his thesis is the higher percentage of dark-skinned individuals who develop autism, which matches those most likely to be at risk for low vitamin D levels. "Much of the disease is iatrogenic, brought on by medical advice to avoid the sun," according to Cannell. "Several types of studies could easily test the theory."[22] Why no studies are under way could be explained by the fact that most studies are funded by pharmaceutical companies, and sunlight can't be patented and sold. Without a government-funded study, we may never know whether his hypothesis is true.

Schizophrenia is another mental illness that's been difficult to understand. It appears that low levels of prenatal vitamin D in the mother do not affect the development of schizophrenia in the child. However, low childhood levels of vitamin D during the years of growth do have some connection to the later development of schizophrenia in adulthood. A Finnish study looked at data for over nine thousand people born in 1966, finding that males who took at least 2000 IU of vitamin D daily during the first year of life were less likely to develop schizophrenia than males who took lower dosages or none at all. Females didn't appear to show a significant association between incidence of schizophrenia and vitamin D supplementation.[23]

Some researchers believe that there's a seasonal effect on the development of both schizophrenia and cognitive performance, depending upon the time of year one is born. Seasonality of birth has been an intriguing way to suggest a link to seasonal sunlight and brain development. Of course, the fetus isn't exposed to sunlight before birth, but the mother's levels of vitamin D circulating in the bloodstream, as well as effects of melatonin (a hormone from the pineal gland of the brain) affect the fetus during the development of brain cells. Studies show that children born in winter tend to get higher grades and do better on standardized achievement scores in reading, math, and science than those born in the summer. The mother's summer stores of vitamin D would be ample for babies born in autumn and early winter, but likely exhausted by springtime, meaning a baby born in the spring likely has low vitamin D levels.

Seasonality also appears to affect the number of children diagnosed with specific learning disabilities, with a higher number of children born in the summer diagnosed with problems than those born in the winter. An Australian study in 2006 showed winter/spring born children did better on physical and cognitive testing than children born in a summer/autumn group.[24]

Vitamin D and the internal chemical reactions it creates hold immense importance for brain studies, but sunlight exposure also stimulates the brain in many ways. At this time the work appears split between studies of vitamin D or studies of exposure to light and the role of melatonin in the brain. Because light's effect on the brain, and vitamin D's effect on body cells are so entirely different, it's difficult to find relationships between the two. They are both vital for optimal brain development and functioning, however. More discussion of the way light affects brain activity through melatonin appears in chapter 7.[25]

THE GENERATION EFFECT

The effects of vitamin D insufficiency are multigenerational, passing in utero from pregnant women to their offspring, who are born with inadequate levels of vitamin D when their mothers are deficient. Following delivery, an infant's vitamin D status typically is 60 to 70 percent of its mother's level. Low levels in infants due to deficiency in their mothers manifest in an array of pediatric problems, such as seizures, tetany (muscle spasms and tremors), weak dental enamel, rickets, cataracts, and limited growth.[26]

Low levels of vitamin D in pregnant women may affect their offspring years later when those children become adults because low levels in the mother's body may be associated with altered brain development in the fetus. While research in this area is new and more is needed, it appears that vitamin D's ability to control cell growth and replacement of cells as they die is critical.[27] These activities are important to cancer researchers trying to stop cell tumor growth and the spread of cancer cells from one area of the body to another. Brain researchers see the other side of the coin—that vitamin D may be valuable in promoting brain cell proliferation that ensures dying cells are replaced as a child grows, for optimal brain health.

In the 1930s, studies done on children with rickets found they were developmentally delayed in motor skill and cognitive development, but when given vitamin D supplementation, their test scores in both developmental areas improved substantially. That sort of research is impossible to do on children today, because cases of rickets are either identified and treated promptly, or unidentified and therefore ignored. Nevertheless, the implications are clear that adequate levels of vitamin D affect mental and cognitive development as well as other body systems.[28]

Theoretically, a baby's low vitamin D levels before birth imprint cells in ways that don't appear until the brain stops growing in early adulthood, the same point at which schizophrenia usually appears. The idea that vitamin D levels impart functional characteristics on various tissues before birth is new, but studies conducted on the origins of diseases and conditions provide evidence that strongly supports a link. This "critical window" as a child develops in the womb confirms the importance of the vitamin D status of mothers-to-be because it can have health implications for the following generation.[29]

BREASTFEEDING AND VITAMIN D FOR DEVELOPMENT

To compound a deficiency at birth, breastfed infants who aren't given vitamin D supplements fall farther behind in achieving adequate levels. Unless nursing mothers get lots of sunlight and D supplements themselves, their milk simply doesn't contain enough vitamin D for their infant to attain good health.

Breastfeeding without vitamin D supplementation is at the root of the growing number of rickets cases in the United States, where most cases occur among dark-skinned infants, who have higher needs for vitamin D than light-skinned infants. Yet health authorities are reluctant to address the issue of vitamin supplementation because they worry it may make mothers less likely to breastfeed, which is the superior and natural way to nourish infants. Any hint that mothers' milk may not be adequate has kept breastfeeding advocates from sounding the alarm that indeed, many modern women's bodies cannot provide enough nutrients for healthy babies. The mothers, too, need more vitamin D than they are getting. In the past, taking baby outdoors for a sunning in a stroller was common practice, giving mother and child a brief exposure to sunlight. In eighteenth- and nineteenth-century Paris, it was popular to send urban infants to live with wet nurses in the countryside for their first year because they returned healthier than infants who lived in the smoke-filled city.[30]

Again, it's an example of how individual nutrient requirements vary and how no "one-size-fits-all" solution will provide optimum health for everyone. Dark-skinned infants, who require larger amounts of vitamin D in the first place, are significantly undernourished when breastfed without supplements (for either mother or child). Parents of color are simply not being given the information they need to protect their children from vitamin deficiencies. It's an issue of pigmentation—not race—that needs to be addressed if we are to have optimal health for all children in the United States.

VITAMIN D AND CHRONIC ILLNESS

How well the body absorbs vitamin D depends upon the amount of sunlight we are exposed to, the supplements we choose to take or are prescribed, and mineral intake, but once inside the body, utilization of these nutrients depends upon how well the digestive system functions. Absorption of vitamins and minerals occurs in the intestines and can be inhibited for a variety of reasons, such as genetic factors that affect absorption, diseases such as inflammatory bowel disease and celiac disease, pancreatic insufficiency, and chronic kidney failure.[31]

Intestinal disorders as well as medications can inhibit absorption of vitamin D and calcium, too. Inflammatory bowel disease (IBD) is linked to osteoporosis; indeed, 15 percent of those suffering from diagnosed osteoporosis also have IBD. Rates are even higher among the elderly and those who are underweight. Even though people with IBD may be ingesting plenty of calcium and vitamin D in supplement form, it's not being absorbed. To make it worse, the medications for IBD—corticosteroids—have been implicated in accelerating the speed of bone loss. Remember, corticosteroids such as prednisone are used to *flush vitamin D out* of the body in the rare case of vitamin D (cholecalciferol) poisoning. Taking small doses of prednisone regularly will inhibit absorption of vitamin D and your physician should guide you as to how to overcome that side effect of taking corticosteroids.[32]

Like plants, we desperately rely on adequate sunlight, the natural source of vitamin D, to thrive. Like green leaves and their photosynthesis process, the chemical reaction within our bodies after sunlight exposure is critical for our physical development and healthy existence. While rickets and osteoporosis have been clearly linked to low vitamin D levels, they have been the easiest to recognize because they are linked to both growth and aging. And they are clearly exhibited in x-rays, making the connection and treatment response visible and concrete. Other disorders, however, have been more difficult to recognize and accept. Because vitamin D receptors have now been discovered in nearly all body cells and have been shown to be present in most internal systems of the body (e.g., organs, nerves, bones, etc.), a number of diseases appear linked to vitamin D. Inadequate amounts of vitamin D have been associated with a broad array of diseases, including oncological, gynecological, autoimmune, gastrointestinal, metabolic, neurological, endocrine, and cardiovascular disorders.

CANCER

Vitamin D, or sun exposure, is now recognized as a way to actually reduce the risk of many cancers. More than sixteen different types of cancer have been linked to vitamin D levels, with significant evidence pointing particularly to breast, prostate, and colon cancers. Epidemiology, or the study of disease patterns, shows that these particular cancers occur more often at higher latitudes, in those whose occupation gives them less opportunity for sunlight exposure, and in people with low levels of vitamin D in the blood. Studies have also found that women with the highest levels of vitamin D and highest exposure to sunlight have half the incidence of breast cancer compared to those with the lowest exposures, and men who were exposed to more sunlight were less likely to suffer from prostate cancer.[33]

In the past twenty years, researchers have begun to notice the epidemiological link between breast cancer incidence and higher latitude that appeared in North America and elsewhere in the world. Mortality from breast cancer has a definite relationship to sunlight, showing cancer occurrence to be inversely proportional to intensity of sunlight. In other words, women living at higher (or lower, for the Southern Hemisphere) latitudes, at greater distance from the equator, develop breast cancer more often than those living closer to the equator. In fact, it is inversely associated, meaning the number of breast cancer cases increases with each increment away from the equator. The decreasing amount of UV radiation and lowered amounts of vitamin D are thought to be the reason. There is also an inverse relationship with eating fish; the more fish in the diet, the lower the risk of developing breast cancer. The amount of vitamin D and omega-3 essential fatty acids in fish may explain the protective effect. It's not limited to North America, either: one study examined rates of breast cancer across the former Soviet Union, compared to total average annual sunlight, and found patterns of increasing breast cancer incidence in areas as sunlight levels diminished.[34]

Looking at mortality maps showing deaths from specific diseases, it's clear that more breast (and prostate) cancer occurs in the Northeast than in the sunny Southwest, or the Southern states. In New York City, where the sun is negligible (due to latitude, climate, and pollution), the annual death rate for breast cancer is 33 per 100,000 women. In San Antonio, which gets at least one-third more sunshine, annual breast cancer deaths number 22 per 100,000 women. The difference in sunlight—and health—is the lives of 11 women in every 100,000 who get breast cancer. It's impossible to tell how many women in San Antonio, and other sunny climes, *didn't* get breast cancer because their vitamin D levels were adequate. Based on this data, researchers in the Department of Family and Preventive Medicine at the University of California, San Diego, suggest that an intake of 800 IU/day of vitamin D may be associated with enhanced survival rates among breast cancer patients.[35]

Like breast cancer, prostate cancer also occurs more frequently in higher latitudes with lower UV radiation from sunlight. Further, research findings reveal that cancers of the breast and prostate act more aggressively in African

Americans than in Caucasian Americans. Skin pigment and vitamin D may explain why, in the United States, more African American men develop prostate cancer than Caucasian men. Age, skin pigment, and genetics, as well as environmental and dietary factors, are important in determining whether one contracts prostate cancer. In all cases, however, vitamin D can make a difference. Several studies now point out the heightened risk for prostate cancer for men with low vitamin D levels. Men with little sunlight exposure and vitamin D deficiency are more prone to develop prostate cancer at a younger age and it is faster growing, whereas men who get more sunshine and tanned seemed to gain a protective benefit against prostate cancer. Other studies have found vitamin D is important in treating these cancers, resulting in fewer deaths from prostate cancer if vitamin D supplements are part of therapy. Vitamin D applied to prostate cancer cells decreased their proliferation, invasiveness, and how quickly they spread to other areas of the body. Michael Holick and T. C. Chen at the Boston University School of Medicine warn, "Adequate vitamin D nutrition should be a priority for men of all ages."[36]

In 1980, Fredric Garland and Frank Garland, brothers and epidemiologists on the faculty at the University of California–San Diego, were the first to realize that colon cancer followed the same geographic and latitudinal parameters as breast and prostate cancer. The incidence of colon cancer, like breast and prostate cancer, is inversely proportional to the amount of sunlight a region receives. More people die of colon cancer in major cities and rural areas that receive less sunlight. While several studies have shown that calcium acts to prevent colon cancer, it appears to work only when combined with adequate vitamin D to assist the body in calcium absorption. As a protective factor against colon cancer, vitamin D can be either taken as a supplement or gained through sunlight exposure.[37]

Calcium and vitamin D, acting synergistically, seem to protect against colon cancer. Studies show that supplementation with one or the other alone doesn't make a difference, but when adequate amounts of both are present, there is a reduced risk. Taking vitamin supplements only works for those who have higher than average amounts of vitamin D in their blood (see chapter 4). Exercise, too, plays a role in staving off cancer. Studies have shown that breast cancer risk is reduced between 30 and 40 percent for women who are very physically active, compared to those who lead more sedentary lifestyles. Researchers in Poland found that women who participated in physical activities outdoors had lower rates of breast cancer than those who engaged in physical labor or vigorous exercise indoors.[38]

Exercise is beneficial in several disease protocols, perhaps largely because it's often done outdoors, under natural daylight. Studies need to be done comparing the benefits of indoor gym workouts with simply walking in the sunshine. Presently, most arguments about exercising outdoors are based upon the psychological benefits, not physiological changes. People feel good outdoors, but there's little documentation to prove anything. Exercise equipment makers and commercial gyms tout their benefits, but there really isn't an interest group promoting simply walking outdoors. More research is done on the dangers of the outdoors, such as asthma, air pollution, and sunburn, than on the positive aspects. As William Morgan, a researcher at University of Wisconsin–Madison notes, "We don't have adequate controlled studies even on the outdoor experience. We need people sitting on park benches looking out on the environment, or feeding pigeons and the like, and then ask the question, 'what effect does this have?'"[39]

Because colon cancer is the third most commonly occurring cancer in the United States and accounts for about 11 percent of cancer deaths, it makes sense to encourage adults to consume adequate amounts of calcium and vitamin D and to exercise outdoors. Again, vitamin D–fortified milk appears to work as a preventive; a large composite study has shown that colon cancer incidence decreased as liquid milk consumption increased. Consumption of other dairy products didn't show a similar result, likely due to the vitamin D fortification found only in liquid milk. Vitamin D and calcium clearly work in tandem in colon cells, just as they do in bone and muscle cells.[40]

Research on vitamin D treatment of colon cancer cells shows it has a destructive effect on these cells, but only when consumed at such a high level that it inhibits calcium balance in the rest of the body. Once a vitamin D analog is perfected that targets only selected activity, it may be useful as a direct treatment without the side effects in the rest of the body that arise from large amounts of vitamin D.[41]

Ovarian cancer, like breast, prostate, and colon cancer, causes more deaths in higher northern latitudes than southern latitudes. When air pollution is considered as well (because it limits the amount of ultraviolet light reaching the ground), ovarian cancer rates show a similar increase in large cities where sunlight intensity was weakened by air pollution.[42]

Skin cancer, which also corresponds to latitudinal and sunshine models, occurs more often in sunnier regions, the opposite of the cancers discussed here. So while sunlight is essential in protecting against deadly breast, prostate, colon, and other cancers, overexposure can lead to painful and disfiguring cancers on the head and neck, as well as malignant melanoma, most especially for those individuals with light-skin pigment. Melanoma risk makes overexposure to the sun problematic and creates a need for a way to obtain vitamin D without sun exposure. While melanoma incidence is increasing quickly in many developed countries, it makes up a small proportion of total cancer incidence and death figures. The Agency for Research on Cancer compiles worldwide cancer records published by the American Cancer Society and notes that there were 160,000 new cases of melanoma (worldwide) in 2002, and 41,000 deaths from the disease that year. In comparison, there were 10.9 million cases of cancer (of all types) reported for 2002, and 6.7 million deaths from all cancer types. While melanoma is a serious disease, it makes up a small portion of the total cancer burden.[43]

Capturing sunlight by harnessing and targeting the active components of vitamin D for a particular health problem, such as cancer, creates a new frontier in medical research. New medicines created from vitamin D analogs offer promising advantages because they can target particular cell activity and when used in large amounts do not affect mineral balance, creating problematic side effects in calcium metabolism.

DIABETES

Diabetes, a metabolic disorder in which the immune system fails to adequately regulate blood sugar, develops in three forms: during childhood (type 1 or insulin dependent), late in life (type 2, or noninsulin dependent), or during pregnancy (gestational diabetes). Type 2 is most easily regulated through controlling carbohydrates in the diet, while type 1 requires regular injections of insulin. Exactly what causes the destruction of insulin-secreting cells in the pancreas, leading to diabetes, remains a mystery, but laboratory experiments have shown that vitamin D acts to suppress the immune response, reducing the proliferation of cells that trigger the disease. In animals, vitamin D actually prevents development of type 1 diabetes. Promising news about protecting against juvenile diabetes (type 1) comes from research into vitamin D.

Diabetes, like most of the chronic diseases now being linked to vitamin D deficiency, shows a higher incidence at latitudes farther from the equator. Both in the Northern Hemisphere and Australia, the rate is higher as one moves away from the equator, suggesting it is related to the amount of vitamin D the body receives.[44]

It appears that type 1 diabetes is related in some way to a mother's vitamin D levels and the levels reached in infancy. Three studies have linked development of diabetes to deficiency of vitamin D in pregnancy or infancy. Some results have found that the risk of developing diabetes years later is lowered by 80 percent when infants were given 2000 IU per day. If infants are given vitamin D supplements during their first year, they are much less likely to develop type 1 diabetes years later. In 2001, researchers in Finland examined the results of lowering the amount of vitamin D given to infants and how that affected type 1 diabetes rates. Before 1975, Finnish infants were regularly given 2000 IU per day, but when the government lowered supplementation to 1000 IU, and more recently to 400 IU, the incidence of diabetes began increasing. While vitamin D deficiency doesn't cause diabetes, it has some effect on the development and intensity of the condition. Two other trials showed that the progress of type 1 diabetes can be slowed by taking vitamin D supplements soon after the disease is diagnosed.[45]

Studies have also shown that vitamin D acts therapeutically to stabilize blood glucose and insulin levels. Sunlight may do more for the body than stimulate the production of vitamin D; it also promotes the production of a substance called alpha-melanocyte-stimulating hormone, which plays a role in regulating insulin and energy balance. Both are essential to controlling conditions like obesity and diabetes.

MULTIPLE SCLEROSIS

Multiple sclerosis (MS), a chronic disease of the nervous system, appears mostly in young and middle-age adults, and more often in females. It involves an autoimmune response that damages the myelin sheaths surrounding nerves in the brain and spinal cord, thereby affecting the nerves' function. The underlying cause of the nerve damage remains unknown. MS has long been a puzzle because it was one of the first chronic diseases that appeared to be linked to latitude. Studies emerging after World War II found significantly more cases of MS in northern latitudes, but no one knew exactly why. Research into vitamin D since the late 1990s has revealed a link between low sunlight levels, particularly in childhood, and later risk of developing MS.[46]

Research in North America has shown clear latitude relationships between sunlight exposure and MS, and the same is true around the globe. Australian researchers clearly link degree of potential sunlight exposure (latitude) to incidence of MS, finding a fourfold increase in occurrence of MS between the Australian cities of Brisbane (28 degrees south) and Hobart (43 degrees south), where there's a 4.9-fold difference in the amount of winter sunlight available. In Europe, a threefold increase in the incidence of MS cases follows a latitude gradient. A relationship between latitude and increasing incidence of MS has also been reported in China. Low levels of omega-3 fatty acids, important to skin cell health, have been linked to the development of MS, too, because they may affect the skin's ability to generate vitamin D from natural sunlight exposure.[47]

MS is a condition that responds to sunlight and vitamin D. When an individual's vitamin D levels are low, symptoms intensify, and when vitamin D levels are high, symptoms subside. It's not known whether lack of vitamin D actually causes MS, but most individuals who develop MS also have insufficient vitamin D levels. Symptoms of MS intensify during the winter and examination of the lesions in the brain shows they increase during winter months. Vitamin D therapy seems to help alleviate symptoms of MS, as well.[48]

Researchers looked at the results of the Nurses' Health Study, which followed over 92,000 women in the United States from 1980 to 2000. They found that women who regularly took 400 IU or more of vitamin D as a supplement had a 40 percent lower risk of developing MS than women who did not take vitamin D supplements. The findings are significant, giving hope that vitamin D supplements may slow the progression of MS. More research needs to be done, including testing for vitamin D levels in the bloodstream, which the Nurses' Health Study did not consider. Researchers have suggested that vitamin D intake of between 1,300 to 3,800 IU per day might help prevent the disease.[49]

Since MS is an autoimmune disease, the immune system in people with MS begins to destroy its own body's cells, believing them to be invaders. Infection from microorganisms as well as foreign antigens in the form of food allergens can trigger activity of the T helper cells, which respond by creating inflammation. The body's own molecules can be mistaken by the immune system, which sends T cell responses to the "invader," creating a situation where inflammation destroys the body's own cells. Suppressing the T cell response to a supposed invader is essential to preventing or limiting autoimmune diseases. Sunlight, or ultraviolet radiation, suppresses the T cell activity in the immune system, thereby diminishing inflammation. It appears that vitamin D or sunlight exposure can mediate the T cell response, reducing the hypersensitivity and down-regulating, or stopping, the T cell assault against the body's own tissues. Sunlight also suppresses melatonin secretion, which triggers responses in T cells. Again, new research points to the importance of sunlight exposure and vitamin D to a developing fetus because immune system tolerances develop before birth.[50]

CHRONIC PAIN

One in six Americans experiences chronic pain, which costs the nation a total of $120 billion a year in medical costs and lost productivity. For some, the source of pain comes from a specific injury, say, to the spinal cord as a result of trauma. But for others, the source of pain is much more elusive. A recent large study done at the Mayo Clinic in Minnesota found that deficiency in vitamin D was associated with persistent, nonspecific muscle and bone pain. In a group of people suffering from chronic generalized pain (none of them were elderly or housebound), 90 percent tested deficient for vitamin D. The researchers concluded that people experiencing chronic pain with no apparent cause for it should be tested and treated for vitamin D deficiency. The condition is often misdiagnosed as fibromyalgia or other diseases, and is characterized by muscle pain throughout the body, joint pain, and deep bone pain. People with the disorder have a loss of muscle strength, too. Further, the pain doesn't respond to analgesics, opiate derivatives, or antidepressants—treatments that are typically effective for other types of pain. The people in the study had been under their physicians' care for the pain, using various over-the-counter and prescription pharmaceuticals, but nothing had worked. When given doses of ergocalciferol (vitamin D_2), their pain and muscle weakness stopped.[51]

Other studies have found that chronic lower back pain is related to vitamin D inadequacy, too. A surprising finding in one study was that younger people with back pain were more vitamin deficient than older persons. And over half of the women of childbearing age in the study had severely deficient levels of vitamin D. The patients had been receiving extensive medical care for a period of time, but no one realized that lack of sunshine or vitamin D was related to their chronic pain. As a result, the study recommended that "screening all out-patients with such pain for hypovitaminosis D [low D levels] should be standard practice in clinical care." They concluded that a large trial of prescription vitamin D as therapy for persistent nonspecific pain is urgently needed.[52]

GROWING PAINS

An increasingly common complaint voiced by children is chronic and nonspecific leg pain. Affecting one in three youngsters between four and six years of age, it is typically labeled and dismissed as normal "growing pains," but these pains have nothing to do with growing. They may occur in clinically normal young children in the middle of the night, causing intense pain for up to fifteen minutes in both legs. The suggested treatment is with ibuprofen or acetaminophen, and reassurances are given to the parents that there's nothing serious to worry about.[53]

Evidence suggests, though, that such pain may indicate the beginning stages of rickets brought about by a vitamin D deficiency. The fact that the incidence of reported growing pains shows the same latitudinal pattern as other vitamin D/sunlight–related conditions is the first clue to a connection. Because there are no valid explanations for children's "growing pains," and because chronic pain and musculoskeletal problems have been linked to vitamin D and mineral metabolism, studies should be pursued to link the two, leading to increased emphasis on children's adequate intake of sunshine and minerals. While that seems logical, in light of the new research being done, it hasn't become widely accepted.

A recent study in Australia linked growing pains in children to muscle fatigue, anatomical differences such as flat feet or knock-knees, and emotional or psychological problems—ignoring the role of vitamin D and minerals in muscle function. Identifying emotional or psychological factors to explain an underlying condition—chronic pain—is confounded by the fact that the parents focused on the child's behavior, which was often characterized by an overall negative mood, aggression, anxiety, and hyperactivity. Certainly, intense pain in the lower legs that doesn't subside, returns mostly at night, and deprives a child of restorative sleep would contribute to negative behavior.[54]

The anatomical differences leading to flat feet and knock-knees are significant to the growing pains syndrome and link directly to vitamin D deficiency and rickets. But too often, the reasoning stalls before the link to vitamin D is made, and the leg pain is treated with pain relievers and not sunlight. That Australian children are increasingly suffering from leg pain should be no mystery: the government there launched an intense and pervasive campaign against skin cancer by admonishing everyone to stay out of sunlight unless swathed in sunscreen. Clearly, the results are coming in as Australian children exhibit increasing "growing pains."[55]

What's particularly distressing in this whole picture of "growing pains" in children is that while pain in adults is recognized and treated, in children it's considered differently. Diagnosing pain is difficult for physicians, mainly because it's a "poorly named, nebulous entity that can be diagnosed only by exclusion," according to pediatrician H. A. Peterson.[56] No test or guidelines exist to help physicians accurately identify growing pains; the diagnosis is often made simply because they can't name a better reason for children's complaints. Growing pains are often confused with juvenile rheumatoid arthritis, which has also been linked to low vitamin D levels in adults. Indeed, as noted in the *American Family Physician*, "When known disorders are excluded, growing pains may represent syndromes that have not yet been identified."[57]

One West Virginia pediatrician discovered that juvenile primary fibromyalgia syndrome (JPFS) was often misdiagnosed as growing pains (20 percent of the time), hysteria (7 percent), and psychological problems (7 percent). JPFS is a relatively common pediatric rheumatologic problem, accounting for 7.5 percent of new diagnoses made by pediatric rheumatologists in the United States. The incidence in Mexico among schoolchildren is only 1.3 percent. New links between fibromyalgia and vitamin D levels should extend to examining how inadequate vitamin D levels affect children and whether "growing pains" are actually leg cramps caused by inadequate levels of vitamin D or minerals.[58] With additional research into the connection between children's leg pain complaints and the onset of rickets, a reliable, noninvasive predictor or indicator of declining bone health could be developed. The old-fashioned idea that children in pain are merely experiencing growing pains needs to be revised.[59]

OBESITY

No one mentions the "sunlight diet," but getting adequate amounts of sunlight keeps people thin. Sunlight stimulates the production of alpha-melanocyte, a hormone that acts to regulate energy metabolism. It works in the brain to regulate insulin and appetite. In lieu of sunlight, supplemental vitamin D seems to help keep weight off. Studies have shown a strong connection between weight gain and sunlight exposure or vitamin D levels. In fact, physicians could just as well take a patient's vitamin D levels as an indicator of their weight before even putting them on the scales. In 2003, a large study (of nineteen thousand people) funded by the Norwegian government found that vitamin D levels were directly related to weight. Those who had the lowest levels of vitamin D were the fattest, with the highest body mass index (BMI).[60]

Calcium, too, plays a role in fat metabolism, and a spate of recent studies link calcium intake from dairy products with weight loss. While the studies have been intriguing, the link between consuming dairy products and calcium as a weight loss agent are hazy, because the studies don't recognize that the milk consumed was fortified with vitamin D. In light of the strong connection to vitamin D found in the Norwegian study, it's unclear whether the weight loss in the calcium studies was due to the calcium or to increased vitamin D consumption in milk. While calcium is essential and dairy products can be part of a healthful diet, the bulk of the findings supporting calcium from dairy products as a weight-loss program were done by groups linked in some way to the dairy industry. The Norwegian study found no direct correlation between calcium intake and BMI. In fact, the researchers actually found a positive association between calcium intake and weight gain for men.[61]

The role of vitamin D and calcium in weight management is fascinating and still not completely understood. Right now theories abound, and all are complicated by the role that the parathyroid hormone plays in fat metabolism. Parathyroid hormone (PTH) and vitamin D both play a part in fat storage, as we saw in chapter 4. While it appears that high levels of vitamin D coincide with being thinner, high levels of PTH are linked with being fatter. High PTH levels and low vitamin D levels are found together. Calcium and vitamin D both act to lower PTH levels, whether alone or together. So if PTH controls weight gain, keeping levels low with adequate amounts of vitamin D might keep the pounds off.[62]

HEART DISEASE

Cardiovascular disease is a leading killer in the United States, and it will come as no surprise that this disease, too, correlates with hours of sunlight exposure. People who experience a heart attack have been found to have lower blood levels of vitamin D at all times of year, compared to control groups. The low point for stored vitamin D levels comes in winter and early spring, which is also the time when most heart attacks occur. This is particularly true in low-sunlight countries like Britain, while areas in the Alps that receive more UV light have a lower incidence of heart disease. The low rate of cardiovascular disease among Inuit people in the Arctic can be explained by the large amounts of vitamin D–rich foods they consume, such as fish and seal meat. When they switch diets to more processed foods, their cardiovascular systems suffer.

Although vitamin D is essential for cardiovascular health, there are concerns that excess vitamin D may be linked to calcification, inflammation, and impaired elasticity in arterial walls because of its activity in metabolizing calcium. But there's no solid connection—the published research data regarding a vitamin D risk factor for atherosclerosis (hardening of the arteries) and heart disease is conflicting. Studies do show a link between vitamin D deficiency due to lack of sunlight exposure and the development of peripheral arterial disease (PAD). PAD results in plaque buildup in the arteries, leading to atherosclerosis. There is also an inverse relationship between vitamin D levels and heart attacks, with lower levels of vitamin D coinciding with increased heart attack risk. Why this is true is unclear at present. Vitamin D provides a protective barrier against PAD because it lowers blood pressure, and an inverse relationship between levels of vitamin D in blood tests and coronary artery calcification has been found.[63] Researchers are uncertain how vitamin D influences calcification in the arteries, however.

Another health paradox may provide the answer to why higher vitamin D levels seem to ameliorate or prevent coronary artery calcification. It appears that osteoporosis occurs coincidentally with calcification of the arteries. A study of elderly women in Denmark found that demineralization in the hip due to osteoporosis was clearly linked to heart disease. The researchers concluded that severe osteoporosis in the hip could be used as an indicator of advanced atherosclerosis and of increased risk for not only hip fracture, but also for coronary heart disease. How it happens is unclear—the calcium being pulled from the bones may be deposited in the arteries, or dietary calcium may be misdirected to arterial muscle tissue rather than to the bones. In either case, inadequate vitamin D levels are likely playing a major role. Supplemental vitamin D seems to lower calcification of the arteries that occurs in 90 percent of coronary artery lesions. Animal studies have shown increasing evidence that arteriosclerosis is an inflammatory condition that can be suppressed by vitamin D in the bloodstream.[64]

HYPERTENSION, OR HIGH BLOOD PRESSURE

Regular exposure to sunlight reduces blood pressure while increasing the amount of vitamin D in the blood. One part of the sunlight spectrum, UV-B light, can also come from artificial sources, such as tanning beds. In one study a group of women with mild high blood pressure was treated with UV-B light and another with UV-A light, both from tanning beds. The UV-A group didn't respond, but the UV-B group showed lower blood pressure and higher vitamin D levels. Not all tanning beds provide UV-B, however, so people relying on tanning beds for vitamin D supplementation should be aware of the type of lightbulbs being used. A less risky option is simply going outdoors for twenty minutes in fall, spring, and summer, which can also lower blood pressure, while building vitamin D stores for winter. (Don't stop taking blood pressure medication because you begin sun exposure—discuss it with your physician.)

Vitamin D is clearly a vital and essential element our bodies manufacture with the help of sunlight. While it appears integral to many of our body's functions, we seem to have discovered only the tip of the iceberg as we begin to understand how it works. While over a thousand vitamin D analogs (vitamin D extracts, you might call them) have already been created, there's plenty of work to be done on what appears to be a budding new frontier of medicine. Understanding exactly how sunlight and vitamin D affect our bodies and our health promises to open up new possibilities for healthier futures and a way to curb the misery from chronic disease.

But vitamin D isn't something just infants and the elderly need worry about. Young women, those least likely to be identified as a chronic disease group, have serious problems without adequate vitamin D. In fact, low vitamin D levels can create a life-or-death situation for many young women around the world when they are ready to give birth. The next chapter looks at this unexamined problem.

Chapter Six

CANARIES IN THE COAL MINE

lothing, housing, diet, and other lifestyle choices are all cultural constructs that reflect our social status and impact our health, and culture is the single greatest determinant of who goes into the sun and who does not. Women, much more than men, have historically and culturally spent more time indoors. The relationship between women and sunlight varies across cultures and groups, but typically women's roles remain within their social norm. It's safer, more comfortable, and easier to do housekeeping, food preparation, and childcare indoors, in privacy and protected from the elements. With modern conveniences, it seems sensible to stay indoors with central air and heat, pleasant lighting, and cozy surroundings; but contemporary women may not realize just how *much* time they spend inside. In the last century we've distorted our environment significantly by turning it into a comfortable, well-lit place, but that's not optimal for our health. No one thinks about it much, but in the long-term scheme of things we may be setting ourselves up for trouble.

SWATHED IN CLOTHING

Clothing may seem insignificant as a risk factor for chronic health conditions, but it plays a significant role. Climate is important, of course, allowing people in warm regions to go without much clothing, soaking up sun as their bodies convert it to ample amounts of vitamin D. On the other hand, cold regions necessitate covering up, making it even more difficult to get sufficient natural vitamin D in areas receiving less ultraviolet radiation (high altitudes, where the sun's rays are more intense, are an exception). Certainly clothing is a sensible solution to the cold, but protection from the elements is only one of the multiple roles clothing plays. Clothing fills needs for group identification, religious affiliation, ethnicity, and status. For such reasons, people living in equatorial zones have sometimes adopted clothing ill suited to the environment, much to the detriment of their health. When culture intercedes, latitude has less influence. Even in sunny Miami, urban Hispanic women have a high prevalence of poor vitamin D status; skin pigment and indoor lifestyles can create a vitamin D "winter" no matter where one lives.[1]

Some Muslim women follow cultural and religious dictates requiring them to cover most of their body when going outdoors or in public—sometimes peeking out through netting inserts in heavy veils. Veiling has little to do with protection from the weather; it is entirely rooted in culture. With such constraints, veiled women seldom get any sunlight on their skin. In the United Kingdom, studies show Muslim women from India, Pakistan, and Bangladesh have extremely low vitamin D levels. Indeed, 85 percent of the women tested had vitamin D levels below 8 ng/ml, while only 3.3 percent of the non-Asian population had levels that low. (As we saw in chapter 4, experts now suggest levels of 60 to 80 ng/ml are optimal.) As a result of such inadequacy, vitamin D deficiency has resurged as a public health concern among the young children of these women. Their children experience rickets and tetany-related seizures.[2]

While several studies have addressed the problem of vitamin D deficiency in Muslim immigrants to northern Europe, it's been difficult to get health statistics from their homelands. Researchers in Saudi Arabia and Lebanon, both sunny locations, found residents had very low levels of vitamin D despite the low latitude. In Lebanon, a study of schoolchildren found only 12 percent had adequate calcium intake (and boys got more than girls) and 16 percent received enough vitamin D. Poverty was a major factor in adequate diet in that study.[3]

In Riyadh, Saudi Arabia, rickets is appearing in children, possibly linked to deficiencies in their mothers, as Saudis of all ages appear to be deficient in vitamin D. Researchers point to several Saudi lifestyle factors: avoidance of sunlight, a dusty atmosphere that may shield residents from ultraviolet rays, and a vegetarian-based diet. Diets high in vegetables and phytates (from grain) don't include adequate vitamin D sources and put all racial/ethnic groups that adopt them at risk for vitamin D deficiency. Saudis, like many Indo-Asian people, eat vegetarian-based diets, consuming only 55 IU/day of dietary vitamin D—about one-seventh of the recommended level.[4]

A 2005 study in northern India revealed that deficiency in vitamin D is widespread and problematic for women and infants there. Blood tests of 207 pregnant women found 84 percent of them with very low vitamin D levels. They also lacked adequate calcium.[5]

HOMEBOUND

Along with dietary supplements, Saudi researchers recommended the redesign of housing to allow more sunlight exposure. In traditional homes across the Indo-Asian region, gardens and sunning areas in the house's central courtyard provide a private area where families can go bareheaded in the sun. Custom dictates women remain indoors, but indoors always included an "outdoors," too, if one could afford it.[6]

Anthropologist Erika Friedl spent years studying women in Iranian villages, where traditional housing patterns provided even secluded women opportunities for sun exposure because they did most of their cooking outdoors on verandas or on rooftops, where they could work without a veil but still be technically within the purdah system. They spent most of their time outdoors in communal (female-only) courtyards or on the verandas, where they carried out their domestic chores, including laundry, food preparation, weaving at looms, and tending children. As villagers modernized or moved to the city, they adopted detached single family–type homes with more modern designs and indoor kitchens. Modern urban apartments and single-family homes allow women little opportunity to do their daily tasks outdoors. All work is centralized inside, where electrical amenities (refrigerators, cooking ranges, and air-conditioning) replace the traditional outdoor lifestyle for homebound women.[7]

Indoor living without access to sunlit terraces spells health problems for women living in seclusion, just as it does for Western women who live in apartments and work at computers, dress in leg-covering slacks, and wear foundation makeup with sunscreen. (Most foundation makeup now includes sunscreen, often at very high SPF levels.) In reality, women under purdah and women in Western offices and apartments aren't leading lives that differ very much from the standpoint of exposure to natural sunlight. For both, dietary vitamin D supplements are essential if they are to offset the lack of sunlight.

While wearing veils has long been a Middle Eastern custom, there have been other cultural practices elsewhere in the world that have kept women bound to the home. Foot binding, practiced in China since the Song dynasty (between 960 and 1279 CE), was a deliberate attempt to modify women's mobility so they couldn't venture out and away from home. While it was accepted as a cosmetic condition, and girls' mothers themselves were the ones who did the binding, no one made a connection between how indoor life weakened girls and women and what that could mean over a lifetime.

The practice of binding feet to make them tiny developed as a way to create and emphasize social class distinctions. Women were valued because they couldn't walk naturally—a sign they were not meant to labor in the field. The families of elite men expected daughters-in-law to have tiny feet, so girls' mothers did all they could to prepare them, wrapping the growing feet so tightly that the bones sometimes fractured as the young girl endured years of pain. *The Good Earth* by Pearl S. Buck provides a glimpse into the social factors involved in binding girls' feet as a way to signify status compared to the feet of rude peasant women who labored in the fields. Bound feet not only symbolized a dependent female, but one who had avoided the outdoors. Her disfigured feet reassured her husband's family she wasn't about to wander off independently or even leave the home.

Foot binding literally bound a woman to the house her entire life. Unable to walk properly, she relied on servants to go to market and do all the chores, and she couldn't enjoy walking in a natural setting. Women shielded their faces with umbrellas if they did go into the sunlight, abhorring tanned skin—another mark of a peasant. For a wealthy family, small indoor gardens and fountains and sunlit courtyards provided the only opportunity for exposure to natural sunlight.[8]

CHILDBIRTH AND VITAMIN D

The cultural covering and secluding of women (deliberately or inadvertently) makes their health fragile—indeed, their shorter stature and increased skeletal fragility as they age directly result from living without enough sunlight. Without adequate vitamin D and calcium as they grow, little girls' bodies don't develop and mature properly for giving birth. A dramatic and deadly consequence of vitamin D deficiency affects pregnant women when their compromised bone development leaves them with a narrow pelvic bone structure—and a baby trapped in the womb.

Historically, dying in childbirth was of great concern to women because once labor began there were few options. The Chinese women's experiences that Buck wrote about clearly reveal the dangers women faced when they grew to adulthood without adequate sunlight and calcium. Buck contrasted the easy birthing experiences of O-Lan, who grew up as a peasant, compared to her more refined daughter-in-law, who was raised differently. The younger woman, whose wealthy parents ensured her feet were bound early, suffered from the common condition of a narrow pelvis due to a lack of sunlight. The main character, Wang Lung, worries while his daughter-in-law's painful labor continues, "My first grandson is about to be born and it is a heavy labor for the mother, who is a town woman and too narrowly made . . ."[9] In the past, high mortality rates due to childbirth were apparently common among the privileged class in China.[10]

While the Chinese experience came earlier in history than the rise of industrialism in the Western world, the results were the same: when girls and women lack minerals and adequate sunlight to make vitamin D, their pelvic bones don't develop properly to give birth naturally. As industrialism swept Europe and North America, children worked long hours indoors, often from dawn to dusk, seldom seeing natural sunlight. Girls spent their hours indoors at looms, or left rural homes to work in urban factories. Dark tenements, factory work, and long sunless days created girls with weakened skeletons, much like the sequestered females in China. Girls in such conditions failed to develop proper pelvic structures, and their rickets during childhood led to difficult childbirth later in life.

Today, as more women around the world adopt indoor jobs and lifestyles and eat mineral-poor diets, the number of babies delivered by cesarean section is increasing quickly around the globe. Half a million women die in childbirth each year and the most significant cause of maternal mortality is obstructed labor. Death in childbirth because the mother cannot vaginally deliver the child amounts to about 410 women for every 100,000 live births worldwide, a figure British researchers remind us is comparable to what it was thirty years ago. And, for many women who do survive a protracted and difficult labor, uncontrollable passage of urine and feces through the torn vagina can disable them for life. Clearly, our technology and our advanced healthcare systems haven't been able to deal with the relatively simple problem—increasing exposure of sunlight or the taking of vitamin D supplements.[11]

In wealthy Western countries, giving birth seems to be something women and their obstetricians have total control over. Options such as birthing chairs, family birthing centers, homey décor in delivery rooms, and even aromatherapy and music create a calm, pleasant experience for women. But in some ways things haven't changed much at all—once labor begins, it's imperative to get the baby out of the womb as quickly as possible. Difficulty and delay can rupture the uterus, or cause birth defects when the baby loses oxygen. Pushing the baby through the birth canal and into the world safely is a process that depends completely on the mother's muscles and pelvic bone structure. Dystocia, the medical term for obstructed labor, happens when a baby's head is too large to pass through the birth canal. Overly large babies may at times be the reason, but the major cause is narrowly formed pelvic bones, due to poor nutrition in childhood and adolescence. That's where calcium and vitamin D play a major role. It's also a major reason why cesarean deliveries are becoming far more common.[12]

Cesareans were never popular and were rarely successful at saving the lives of mothers or infants. Forceps, invented in the seventeenth century, aided difficult deliveries. An awkward tool, it put men in control of childbirth, relegating midwives to the sidelines. The forceps may have saved some infants' lives, but it often damaged both babies and their mothers. Further, the tool could not overcome the restrictions of a physically narrowed pelvis.

Cesarean surgical deliveries became more common as industrialization, urbanization, and hospitals created both a need and a possibility for surgical childbirth. Anesthesia, which appeared just prior to the American Civil War, made cesareans more practical. Cesarean surgery wasn't like amputation, which was done with speed while the patient was held in place. A cesarean was complicated, time consuming, and extremely risky. Infection and blood loss were still major dangers, however, and for almost a century (1787 to 1876) not a single woman survived a cesarean in Paris.[13]

Modern cesarean surgery developed in the American South as a way to save slave women's lives—and owners' investments. Louisiana was a leading state in the number of cesarean sections before the Civil War, all of them performed on slaves. Slave women often had difficult labors and those who survived frequently suffered from internal injury the rest of their lives.

Young black women frequently died in their first labor, and while there are many reasons why a slave woman in the antebellum South might have been in poor health, the cause of obstructed labor was always the same: the mother's pelvis was too narrow. Other factors play a role, but for most, pelvic shape, like the rest of the skeleton, depends on obtaining minerals and sunshine as one grows to maturity. Certainly nutrition played a part in quite literally shaping young slave bodies. These young girls no doubt received inadequate diets, which led to distorted and narrowed pelvic structures. Slave diets were low in calcium and magnesium, while minerals were excreted from the body through perspiration during long hours of work in the warm climate. Not all slaves worked in the fields and were therefore receiving ample sunshine. Many worked indoors, doing laundry, cooking, or engaged in light manufacturing.

Because owners saw them as an investment—indeed, one that paid dividends when bearing new slave children, medical care was important. In the 1850s, Dr. James Marion Sims, dubbed the "father of American gynecology," established himself at the Woman's Hospital in New York City after a decade of experimental surgery on Southern slave women who suffered the aftereffects of very difficult labor and delivery. Sims, as well as other medical colleagues throughout the South, practiced on a steady stream of injured slave women who survived their first pregnancy, but were internally damaged for life.[14]

Sims began experimenting on slave infants suffering from tetany, a condition related to inadequate vitamin D that results in seizures, inability to nurse, and eventual death. It was a well-known condition among enslaved families, but at the time no one knew what caused it. Sims attributed it to slave mothers' ignorance and to laying babies on their backs in cradles. Often mistaken for tetanus, an infectious reaction to bacteria, tetany appeared as an infantile form of rickets, evidenced by seizures and as craniotabes, with skull softening and late closure of the fontanel, or the traditional soft spot on the top of a baby's head. Sims thought the skull plates had shifted out of position, and he perfected his unique technique for "curing" such infants by inserting a shoemaker's awl into the skull and using pressure to pry the occipital and parietal bones into place. Survival rates were low, but eager for recognition within the medical profession, he published several articles in the mid-1840s on the technique in the *American Journal of the Medical Sciences*, garnering a mixed reception.[15]

For their white masters, slave babies had little value: they required several years of feeding and care before they could work. Their mothers, however, were investments. "By the early nineteenth century, slave women were clearly recognized as so-called breeders," notes historian Deborah Kuhn McGregor. "Their ability to reproduce became central to their worth as property to the master."[16]

Confounding the situation was the high incidence of rickets among poorly fed slave children, particularly girls. Rickets led to deformities of the pelvis and difficult childbearing, often resulting in death during a young woman's first labor. Survivors were left with internal damage as pressure on the birth canal created leaking tears in the bladder or rectum, known as vesicovaginal fistula. It was a common occurrence and left women unable to bear children, perform work, or retain any shred of dignity due to incontinence of bladder and/or bowel.

In 1845, Sims began experimenting with surgical techniques to repair fistulas on slave women in a backyard cabin-clinic beside his Montgomery, Alabama, home. Before anesthesia, he used opium to help the women endure multiple surgeries, operating on one woman named Anarcha thirty times. He eventually perfected his technique and moved to New York City, where he could develop a wider practice, leaving slave women behind.[17]

After moving north to Women's Hospital, Sims had scores of impoverished, malnourished Irish immigrant women to work on, who also suffered from skeletal development inadequate for childbearing. The potato famine had forced them out of Ireland and into dark urban tenements. Life in pastoral agricultural settings, consuming dairy products, and getting plenty of sunlight disappeared as a surge of immigrants moved to industrial cities in both the United States and Europe. Just as rickets became a scourge of the cities, so did obstructed labor, as the girls with misshapen skeletons grew up to have babies. Until cesarean surgery was perfected, patching up injuries from difficult labor was the best response for those women who survived childbirth with a contracted pelvis.

Eventually, antiseptics and anesthesia (and antibiotics after World War II) made cesarean sections successful and the number of surgeries grew. Physicians began using the technique sooner, before women were exhausted from long labor and the fetus was overstressed or without oxygen. Performing a cesarean earlier in labor became controversial in the medical community, but it saved more mothers and infants. The rate of cesarean sections soared, leveling off a bit in the years after World War II, when emphasis on vitamin D–fortified milk and daily doses of cod liver oil may have helped that generation of girls when they came of age to bear children.

THE CESAREAN EXPLOSION

Dying in childbirth seems part of a very long-ago era, a hazard of life in days gone by. Today, with a myriad of technologies that allow monitoring of the fetus from implantation through delivery, the idea of a mother dying during childbirth seems remote. Yet, it's not as rare as it should be. In fact, childbirth-related deaths threaten many of the world's women who lack access to surgical delivery as well as the proper diet and lifestyle to eliminate the need for it.

Since 1987, the World Health Organization (WHO) has been working to reduce maternal mortality; their challenge is to eliminate deaths from obstructed labor (dystocia), which is a killer of both mother and child. In developing countries, obstructed labor is one of the five major causes of maternal deaths, with a death rate of up to five women per one thousand live births. Poor nutrition for growing girls is the cause of obstructed labor, but lack of medical facilities for surgical deliveries exacerbates the number of deaths. And the need is growing. In 1998, researchers at an international meeting on Maternal Mortality in the Developing World warned that obstructed labor is one of the most common preventable causes of death among mothers and their babies in developing countries, and they outlined prevention policies that should include discouraging early motherhood in young women (many of whom are under sixteen years old) and improving nutrition for females "during infancy, childhood, early adulthood, and pregnancy." Too often, early motherhood occurs before a girl's body is fully developed, before pelvic bones are fully grown. Rickets and osteomalacia (weakened bone structure) make the condition even worse. Nutritional deficiencies in calcium, vitamin D, folic acid, iron, and zinc cause most of the incidents of obstructed labor worldwide.[18] A flat pelvis, through which a baby's head cannot pass, is related to the mother's height, which directly corresponds to nutritional status in childhood and adolescence, according to Justin Konje and Oladapo Ladipo, British obstetrics professors.[19]

The rising number of cesarean sections is of concern to health authorities worldwide because third-party payers—insurance companies and governments—are seeking ways to cut the increasing number of expensive surgeries. In the United States, the rate of cesarean deliveries has steadily increased from 9.1 percent of all live births in 1974 to 21.2 percent in 1984 to 31.1 percent as of 2006—an increase of over 40 percent since 1996. A rising trend worldwide has also been documented across cultures and in both developing and wealthier nations.[20]

Dystocia, due to a small or flattened pelvis, plays a major role in deciding whether to perform cesarean surgery as well as the need for surgical deliveries for subsequent births, because the uterus has been weakened with the initial cesarean section and can't withstand vaginal delivery. Therefore, part of the statistical increase in cesareans is from women having additional children, which are often delivered by cesarean section as well, which makes up about a third of the total number of cesareans performed.[21]

It's difficult to grasp just how important of a concern the occurrence of obstructed labor is in the United States and worldwide, because in most cases it's a subjective condition. The obstetrician relies on his or her personal judgment of the woman's condition before and during labor. It's not something easily codified or determined with a blood test or x-ray. In some cases, a four-day-long labor is not considered long enough to perform a cesarean; in other cases a consultation between physician and the expectant mother beforehand leads to a scheduled cesarean before labor begins. The medical community as well as maternal advocacy groups find it a difficult topic to grasp, largely due to the differing opinions about when to end a difficult natural labor by proceeding with a surgical intervention. Theoretically, through improved prenatal care, women who may encounter difficulty due to pelvic structure would be alerted to the problem by their obstetrician before labor even begins, and cesarean section would be agreed upon without subjecting the mother and baby to an unnecessary and difficult labor.

Because a precise diagnosis of dystocia is lacking, determining how many needless cesareans are performed becomes a hypothetical argument. Nevertheless, the Centers for Disease Control (CDC) and a vanguard of anticesarean advocates are currently focused on decreasing the number of cesarean deliveries. One strategy is to challenge the accepted practice of following an initial cesarean section with operative deliveries for all subsequent births. Because cesarean surgery weakens uterine muscles and can be a risk factor in later vaginal deliveries, obstetricians have usually opted for cesareans following an initial cesarean delivery. By getting more women who already had a cesarean section to deliver a subsequent baby vaginally, the overall rates can be lowered. Yet that is not proving to be best for mother or baby, and is creating additional health and often malpractice issues because the inadequate pelvis problem still exists, creating a dangerous situation for mother and baby during delivery.[22]

Another concern is fetal size. How large a baby is too large for the mother's pelvic structure to deliver safely? In many cases, fetal size is determined by ultrasound results (which is likely to be off by 20 percent). Obstetricians often opt for surgical delivery for babies who are expected to weigh over eight pounds. Whether the mother would have delivered naturally or not, the obstetrician uses his or her judgment to avoid medical complications and ensure a safe and healthy mother and child. Certainly, many of the large babies now delivered by cesarean might have been just fine after undergoing a difficult natural delivery, but there's no way to accurately determine the outcome ahead of time.[23]

So when is a cesarean unnecessary? That's unclear, yet critics of cesarean section come from maternity care advocacy groups, such as Lamaze and the American College of Nurse-Midwives, who abhor cesarean section as an unnecessary medical procedure that eliminates the option for women to deliver babies naturally. Those groups see cesareans as creating unneeded medical risk for the mother during surgery, but they are not addressing the reasons for cesareans. Literature and materials from such groups seldom mention *why* cesareans are performed or the need for prevention. Adequate minerals and vitamin D during girls' developmental years could prevent many cases of dystocia—and therefore cesareans—when women face delivery.

Viewing cesarean section as an unnecessary procedure forced upon unsuspecting pregnant women by obstetricians and surgeons ignores the real problem. Claims from groups such as the Coalition for Improving Maternity Services include the statement, "Healthy women, who should rarely need operative delivery, undergo a large percentage of the cesarean sections performed in the US." Yet, what is the definition for "healthy women"? Everyone in the debate, which at bottom is an issue of medical risk, expensive surgery, and who shall pay, ignores prevention: the health and nutrition status of growing girls.[24]

In the end, it does come down to the bottom line. Cesarean deliveries can cost more than twice as much as natural deliveries and require twice as long a hospital stay for the mother. Both the federal government and health insurance companies are intent on forcing down the number of cesarean sections performed each year, hoping to eliminate what the CDC believes to be unnecessary expenses for healthcare. They claim that by pushing the number of cesareans down by 8 percent in 1991, over a billion dollars in physician fees and hospital charges could have been eliminated. Today, in US hospitals, a cesarean section is 130 percent to 200 percent higher in cost than a normal vaginal delivery, while the charge for a forceps-and-vacuum delivery (pulling the fetus's head with a suction device) runs only 25 to 30 percent more. The higher costs for the more intensive medical care means cesarean sections add $5.5 billion to US healthcare costs annually. Health insurance companies would like to see more forceps-and-vacuum deliveries, but physicians are wary of how that affects their patients, the babies, and ultimately their own malpractice insurance rates.[25]

Today's mothers also must deal with insurance companies that refuse to cover them once they have given birth via cesarean section. Because after an initial cesarean delivery, subsequent births are more likely to result in cesarean surgery as well, insurance companies refuse to cover such women. While group coverage sponsored by employers doesn't reject such cases, it becomes a problem when women in some states try to buy individual insurance plans. States vary in regulating whether insurance companies must cover "preexisting conditions," health conditions that may reappear and cost money for treatment. States also vary in whether they allow cesarean delivery to be considered a reason for exclusion, or whether it falls under any special rules. Sometimes the insurance carrier includes a "rider," a stipulation saying coverage for cesarean delivery is excluded for a certain period of time from when the applicant began the coverage. In some cases, applicants are accepted by an insurer but must pay additional premiums or higher deductibles if they have had prior cesareans. For some companies, a woman who has had a prior cesarean may be covered only if she has been sterilized since the cesarean or is over age forty. Adding further to the problems women needing cesareans encounter is that once they have been denied coverage from an insurance company because they applied and were turned down due to a prior cesarean, they are "red-flagged" in the industry and other insurers may automatically deny them coverage.[26]

While Western nations argue over how to stop the increasing number of cesarean deliveries, in many parts of the world women who desperately need surgical deliveries are not able to get them. Rates for cesareans are rising worldwide, but in places like Nigeria, youth pregnancies for women (ages fourteen to sixteen) and the taboo against cesarean deliveries in a culture where women are shamed if they do not deliver their babies themselves create higher death rates than necessary. In one study, death rates of adolescent mothers were 4,863 per 100,000 live births, with 76 percent of the deaths due to obstructed labor.[27]

There is a controversial surgical alternative to cesarean section that is gaining attention. Symphysiotomy, a surgical procedure abandoned by Western medicine when cesarean section was adopted, may be a solution. In normal pregnancy, hormones (relaxin and progesterone) soften the cartilage linking the pelvic bones at the center to enable bones to spread slightly. In some vaginal deliveries, the joint will separate beyond a normal spreading on its own, causing postdelivery pain and difficulty walking. Symphysiotomy is a minimally invasive surgery that splits the pubic bone apart to allow the baby's head to pass through the pelvis during delivery. The surgical procedure replicates what the body might do naturally, to allow a too-large infant head to pass through the pelvis. A scalpel is inserted through the skin over the pubic symphysis (cartilage joining the left and the right pubic bones), and the joint is cut apart by pivoting movements of the scalpel, cutting through the ligaments. Simple to do, it takes only local anesthesia, gloves, a urinary catheter, and a scalpel. Kenneth Bjorklund at the Karolinska Institute in Stockholm suggests that it may be a simple way to save many young mothers living in areas without access to surgical deliveries. The procedure is simple and can be taught to healthcare providers who aren't necessarily surgeons. No stitches are necessary to close the small incision and chances of infection are minimal.[28]

While symphysiotomies are simple to do, the woman isn't up and about quickly. In fact, she will probably take longer to heal than if a cesarean section was performed because, until the joint heals back together, walking is both difficult and painful. A bladder catheter for a week, along with bed rest and a firm strap across the lower abdomen to hold the pelvis together are all necessary. In some cases (between 2 and 4.6 percent), long-term pain, urinary incontinence (if the procedure is done inaccurately), and difficulty walking can make life miserable.[29]

Do the benefits outweigh the risks? Over the past century, more women survived symphysiotomies than cesarean sections done in the same hospitals. There's less chance for infection and other complications than with cesareans. The rate of infant survival was similar between the two procedures. After a symphysiotomy, the pelvis remains permanently expanded a bit, never growing back together as tightly as it was, making future vaginal deliveries easier.[30]

No one can predict whether symphysiotomy will become an accepted practice or not, but it provides a simple, cheap way to deliver babies for women with inadequate pelvic bones. The long period of convalescence after symphysiotomy is difficult for poor peasant and laboring women to enjoy because they must return to their work quickly and need to walk as soon as possible. Again, like most medical solutions to health problems caused by inadequate nutrition, it's only a stopgap and not a preventive.

NUTRITION = PLANNED PARENTHOOD

Even after a woman stops growing taller, her pelvic bones continue to develop, requiring calcium and vitamin D in order to shape the bony pelvis. Osteomalacia, a weakening of bone structure usually seen as women age, can develop at earlier ages and cause problems with childbirth. Research links the height of the mother to pelvic size; both are related directly to the nutritional status of the woman from childhood. In the United States, women who stand less than five feet one and a half inches (157 cm) tall are likely to have inadequate pelvic bone development and more likely to deliver by cesarean section. Because genetics affect height as well, cutoff points have been identified in different countries. Some examples of height numbers below in which the likelihood of cesarean is high are: 156 cm in Denmark, 150 cm in Kenya, 140 cm in India, and 160 cm in Zimbabwe.[31]

Compounding the problem for women who are poorly nourished in childhood and adolescence is the situation when they immigrate to countries where their diets improve. Immigrant women who began eating more protein and larger amounts of food after their growing had stopped, and those who remained in poor nations but were given improved nutrition and vitamin supplements as part of a prenatal care program had greater risk of obstructed labor. Vitamin D and calcium supplementation given to pregnant women had no effect on enlarging their pelvic bones—they had stopped growing years earlier. If the woman's bone structure and pelvis develop inadequately due to poor childhood nutrition, but while pregnant her nutrition improves, the result is a large baby that can't be born naturally through her narrow pelvic bones.

An interesting argument developed in the early 1990s when researchers at the London School of Hygiene and Tropical Medicine questioned the ethics behind providing nutritional supplements to pregnant women to increase the birth weight of their newborns. In the developed world, prenatal supplements and concomitant larger babies have led to an increase in cesarean deliveries, but in the third world, where access to cesarean deliveries is limited and mothers have inadequate pelvic development due to malnourishment in their youth, larger babies mean more mothers (and babies) dying during labor. Clearly, a smaller baby's head is easier to pull through the birth canal. In fact, several cultural groups worldwide have long practiced limiting pregnant women's food consumption with the goal of limiting the fetus's size in order to avoid difficult births. Interventions from well-meaning health organizations seek to address nutritional shortcomings by giving pregnant women vitamin supplements to avoid low–birth weight babies. That creates larger babies but does not address the mother's inadequate pelvic structure, nor do such programs provide for surgical intervention to deliver the larger babies. While some suggest limiting or abandoning prenatal supplements to avoid birthing problems, it's a catch-22: withholding vitamins and minerals from impoverished mothers can cause birth defects and later problems for the inadequately nourished newborn. At issue as well is the international antimalarial effort in developing countries, which relies on antimalarial medications that result in increased fetal growth. Those medications create a life-threatening situation most pregnant women aren't aware of—and aren't being told about. Without access to surgical deliveries, large babies in the bodies of undernourished young women present an ethical dilemma: should health workers provide supplements or not? It's clear that intervention, with specific goals of increasing fetal birth weight, may actually increase maternal mortality.[32]

The issue has evolved because of the continued malnourishment of young girls. The solution is to provide necessary cesarean surgeries for mothers who need them now, while concentrating resources on improving the nutritional status of little girls who will become the next generation of mothers. Providing calcium and vitamin D during childhood and adolescence will help to eliminate the problem of obstructed labor. By the time women become pregnant, it's too late to undo years of nutrient deficiency.

NEANDERTHAL MAMAS

In the short term, a woman's contracted pelvis seems to be an individual problem. On the larger stage, however, it can affect the population's future. History doesn't usually pay attention to the size and shape of female pelvic bone structure, but it has been significant in determining survival. Some theorists hold that more than one group of early people may have succumbed to extinction because they could no longer give birth to succeeding generations.

In 1829, when the first Neanderthal fossil remains were uncovered in Belgium, they were ignored because no one was ready to interpret them. By the 1860s, however, Neanderthal remains had been discovered at several other sites. In 1864, August Mayer, a German anatomist, offered the interpretation that the thick bones and distinct skull shape of the Neanderthal (enlarged eyebrow ridges and low forehead) were due to rickets. He also suggested that the bones came from a bowlegged Mongolian Cossack who had run off from Russia in 1814, hidden in a cave, and died. Other experts ventured that the remains were those of an ancient Celt or even a member of the ape family. Rudolf Virchow, biologist and founder of medical pathology, examined the remains in 1872 and agreed that the individual had a bad case of rickets but declared that it was not an ancient person. His proclamation silenced the discussion for years.[33]

As more Neanderthal remains were uncovered, they supported the idea that the ancient individuals suffered from poor health. Their decayed teeth, advanced arthritis, and bone malformation from childhood lent support to the theory they had rickets. In 1970, *Nature* published an article about a Neanderthal child with rickets, adding to the body of opinion that European Neanderthals suffered from the disease, likely due to a lack of sunlight and vitamin D.[34]

The Neanderthals moved into Europe before dying out about thirty thousand years ago. It is believed they had drifted north away from central Africa into the higher latitudes and then were pushed southward by plummeting temperatures and moving ice sheets as the climate chilled. Storms, clouds, and lack of sun may have taken a toll.

A team of researchers from the University of Cambridge made up of archeologists, anthropologists, geologists, and climate modelers have come up with a definitive series of maps covering climate change, animal and plant populations, and the paths of human and Neanderthal migration with the seasons. They confirm that plummeting temperatures pushed Neanderthals south from northern Europe about thirty thousand years ago, as ice sheets moved south. Archaeologist William Davies, a member of the team, was surprised at "the extent to which Neanderthals seem to have been deterred by the cold and retreated as the going got tough." The earliest modern humans, the Aurignacians, appeared about forty thousand years ago, and they also had a hard time coping with the stormy weather. They moved down into southern France and along the Black Sea. When the Gravettian people appeared in eastern Europe about the same time that the Neanderthals were making their way south, these Gravettians brought along technology that included fishing nets, textiles, and language, and they survived while the other humanoid populations dwindled to extinction.[35]

Cold, cloudy weather and lack of dietary sources of vitamin D would certainly have weakened Neanderthal health, but there are many factors that determined their fate. Whether or not they suffered from vitamin D deficiency is easier to ascertain. Their large skulls with thick brow lines, combined with short legs, bent spines, and decayed teeth indeed suggest rickets. Anthropologists know that Neanderthals suffered severe cases of arthritis, bone malformation in childhood, and missing teeth. In 1970, experts discovered that several Neanderthal children's skulls revealed severe cases of rickets. If they experienced such widespread vitamin D deficiencies, it's likely that young Neanderthal women were increasingly unable to give birth to the next generation and a large proportion of women probably died in childbirth.[36]

Pelvic remains of Neanderthals are puzzling because they suggest very young women were giving birth, perhaps girls too young to have developed adequate bone structures. The skeletal evidence reveals that the Neanderthal women died while they were of childbearing age, and perhaps the shortage of females became crucial, especially because their overall population levels were low. Anthropologist Ezra Zubrow suggests that a reduction in fertility of 1 percent would have led to extinction of the Neanderthals within a thousand years.[37]

Anthropologist Anne Zeller of the University of Waterloo, Ontario, writes that "since most Neanderthal females appear (on the basis of skeletal evidence), to have died while still of childbearing age, perhaps there was a shortage of Neanderthal females and some of the males did look elsewhere for mates." When young women of childbearing age experience high mortality rates, it doesn't take long to affect a population—perhaps the Neanderthal's demise is partly linked to the effects of inadequate sunlight and bone mineralization.[38]

In the 1990s, Kennewick Man, another major ancient fossil find, this time in Washington State, set off a round of speculation. Kennewick Man was eventually seen to represent a unique type of people who existed in North America about 9,500 years ago but disappeared without a trace. The males lived fairly long lives; the skeletal remains reveal they died between the ages of thirty-two and forty years, with one skeleton being older than fifty.

For women it was a different story. Females died young, between eighteen and twenty-three—in their prime childbearing years. The women were very short in stature and their tiny bones show evidence of annual stress fractures, likely from poor diet during winter. Those people, too, may have died out as girls' nutrition and health could no longer support successful childbearing. A small group of people losing females at an early age simply cannot replenish itself.[39]

The stories of early extinctions are important because, while they are extreme examples, they point out how the future of societies can depend upon the health of young girls. Lack of fossil and skeletal remains showing that women survived beyond the age of initial childbearing spells the end for any group, as the mating pressures brought on by a surplus of men would force immature females into childbirth before their bodies were fully developed. Males, eating a similarly inadequate diet and experiencing the same lack of sunlight (from cloudy climatic conditions), would have simply gotten older—cranky and stiffened from arthritis. Unable to replenish itself with new generations, it wouldn't have taken long for the entire population to disappear.[40]

Sunlight is important to healthy bones, but calcium is also essential. Reinhold Vieth, an epidemiologist at Mount Sinai Hospital in Toronto who has studied vitamin D extensively, suggests that paler skin pigment alone would not have been enough to ensure human survival at northern latitudes. Calcium intake from environmental sources was essential. Sources of calcium such as fish bones are easily consumed after cooking but would have been difficult to eat raw. Until cooking pots and meal preparation technology were invented, dietary sources of calcium were likely minimal. Seafood and bone broths provided calcium once cooking was perfected. It's likely that mineral-laden drinking water was more important to the diet than food sources of calcium.[41]

Examining the relationship between women's health and sunlight is not an entirely bleak story. Drinking water and sunlight, and their link to traditional lifestyles shaped by geography, may explain a medical enigma surrounding the one group of women in the United States who are not facing increasing numbers of cesarean deliveries. Native American women living in the Southwest have the lowest cesarean rates in the country, 9.6 percent, compared to over 27 percent for all US women. While some proponents give credit to the Indian Health Service and its hospital in Santa Fe, New Mexico, it appears there's a significant preventive factor involved. In trying to figure out why Navajo women also experience lower rates of osteoporosis and hip fracture than Caucasians, despite a diet low in calcium, researchers discovered that the mineral content of drinking water in the Four Corners area (high desert where Arizona, New Mexico, Utah, and Colorado meet) supplied most of their calcium needs.[42]

Navajo women drink about two liters of water a day, which when tested showed 212 mg of calcium, 150 mg of magnesium, and 8 mg of zinc. While that's below the minimum calcium recommendation of 800 mg per day (and most American women only consume 600 mg), Navajos may be absorbing it better because their intake is spread throughout the day and other minerals are consumed at the same time. Traditional Navajo cooking also includes generous sprinklings of juniper ash made from burning juniper needles, which is high in mineral content. When juniper ash is added to blue corn meal mush, it provides a whopping 800 mg of calcium per cup, compared to 300 mg/cup of calcium in milk.[43]

Mineral-rich drinking water provides an excellent source of calcium because it's in the form of hydrated ions and more easily absorbed than from food sources. Calcium metabolism in bones appears to be increased by the presence of bicarbonate and silica from drinking hard water, too. A study of over four thousand elderly French women found that the calcium content of mineral water actually resulted in a slight increase in bone density compared to dietary calcium.[44]

In wealthier nations, young girls are reluctant to drink milk, opting to avoid any weight gain during growth years. While fortified milk is an excellent source of calcium and vitamin D, if young women avoid it in the quest for thinness, their bodies will be unprepared for natural childbirth. Rather than exhorting them to drink milk, which they are refusing to do, it might be better to adopt a national health message to drink ample amounts of mineral water and spend time in the sun as a way to strengthen the body and prepare for childbirth.

In closing, it appears that many of the technologies and cultural developments we accepted to make our lives easier and more comfortable may actually not have been very good for us. Electricity, heavy clothing, even water softeners and modern housing all play a part in shielding us from the natural elements so essential to strong bones and bodies. And for young women in many parts of the world, sunlight and minerals can mean the difference between life and death.

Chapter Seven

CIRCADIAN RHYTHMS

While we mainly think of sunlight as a source of vitamin D, it is essential for many other processes in the body, affecting metabolism, neurological functions, even fertility. While much attention (and much of this book) has focused on the intriguing activity of sunlight through its role in creating vitamin D, there is more to discover regarding the global effects of sunlight on human physiology and health.

Sunlight acts as a regulator of our internal clock, which shapes our behavior based on the time of day, of the month, and of the year. The daily cycles of biological processes in plants and animals are known as "circadian rhythms." They are a recurring phenomenon, as shown by their name taken from *circa*—Latin for "around," and *dies*—meaning "day." Other biological cycles react to monthly and seasonal changes in light, the study of which is called chronobiology. The terms—circadian rhythms and chronobiology—are often used interchangeably. About twenty years ago, circadian rhythm research emerged as a major field of medical study, especially in psychiatry. However, interest eventually faded because studies hadn't provided any practical applications or therapies. Now, new frontiers in chemistry and molecular biology have put the field of chronobiology "on the verge of a renaissance," according to one researcher. We understand a bit how the chronobiological system responds to circadian and seasonal rhythms. The growing number of experts working in the field have led some to refer to it as a "clockwork explosion." Understanding how our inner clock functions allows better measurement and treatment protocols, providing real benefits in patient therapy.[1]

A quick overview of how light intensity varies daily and seasonally shows how our circadian relationship with the sun is always in flux. Because the earth is a sphere, sunlight intensity varies with latitude, decreasing incrementally as you move away from the equator. The earth is also tilted at a 23.5-degree angle, which means that as it moves in its annual cycle around the sun, points on the earth's surface receive varying amounts of radiation. Solar radiation is most intense when the sun is directly overhead, something that happens at the equator or in summer at higher latitudes. In the Northern Hemisphere, December 21 (the winter solstice) is when the North Pole has moved farthest from the sun, and when the least amount of solar radiation is available. The opposite happens in the Southern Hemisphere, where midsummer is occurring. At the equator it's always about the same, twelve hours of sunlight and twelve hours of darkness.

At the equator, it's pretty easy for the body to adjust to sleeping and waking rhythm, since they never change. But as you move away from the equator, as many of our ancestors did, things become more complicated because the amount of sunlight is always fluctuating. Every day is different from the one before, as far as natural sunlight goes. Days gradually get shorter, until at a certain point they begin to lengthen, while the night shortens. To make it more problematic, short days are accompanied by the sun sitting low on the horizon, not directly overhead, providing a limited amount of ultraviolet radiation during a shortened period of daylight. Our bodies have to monitor and calibrate to minimal amounts of sunlight in midwinter, then gradually alter until we are functioning during long days with intense sunlight in summer. It's a huge adjustment, but because it's done incrementally and periodically, a rhythm develops. We have evolved to live and act seasonally, turning to eating carbohydrates and fats as fall comes, then sleeping earlier and longer during winter, restoring our energy until spring revives us and we move into summer and very short nights, with far less time to sleep. Our ancestors were like the birds and herds that followed the sun, heading south to sunnier winter homes as the days shortened. We're trying to shift away from that natural pattern as we pursue indoor lifestyles and our bodies react by moving into the natural mode to handle what seems like continual dusk. We adopt a slowed and sometimes lethargic level of activity until the sun returns in force. We're evolving from being a mobile species, dependent upon seasonal migration, to a place-bound existence, dependent upon electrical lighting. And our circadian rhythms are trying to help us adjust.

CIRCADIAN RHYTHMS

Sleeping and waking patterns are determined by the circadian rhythms, which involve activities in the brain, hormone production, and cellular renewal. These are natural rhythms, established by the waxing and waning of sunlight and darkness. Yet they aren't static. When a plant or animal is reared under a regular schedule of artificial light, it eventually adjusts to the new light pattern. But take away the light—artificial or natural—and animals lose their circadian moorings and begin acting in a free-floating manner—sleeping and waking at unrelated intervals. After a time in total darkness, their bodies lose control of their chronobiological systems. They no longer function in a periodic fashion, but sleep randomly, and when awake they are seldom at peak alertness.

In animals and humans, the circadian clock is in the brain, actually in the suprachiasmatic nucleus (SCN) in the hypothalamus, a gland about the size of a walnut located at the underside of the brain at the end of the brain stem. The SCN receives direct input from light receptors in the retina of the eye, telling the brain what the length of the day is. The SCN varies in size with the seasons, becoming twice as large in autumn than in summer, when it is at its smallest point. It changes size coinciding with times when the amount of daylight undergoes its greatest change. The shortening days of autumn and the lengthening days of spring cause the SCN to form more cells. The number of cells in the SCN expands at both the spring and the autumn equinox and diminishes during the summer and the winter solstice, becoming slightly smaller at midsummer than at midwinter.[2]

The pineal gland, located behind the hypothalamus, creates and releases an appropriate amount of melatonin hormone. Melatonin, a natural hormone produced in the pineal gland, eyeball, intestinal tract, and a few other cell sites, circulates throughout the body and regulates circadian rhythms. Levels of melatonin signal the body's autonomic system to become sleepy.

Melatonin levels rise at night and drop during the day. Melatonin production in the pineal gland is regulated by environmental light on a twenty-four-hour cycle. The retina in our eye signals the pineal gland to begin or stop production of melatonin, depending upon the amount of light the retinal photoreceptor cells detect. When it becomes dark, the photoreceptors signal the body to produce norepinephrine, which activates melatonin production. In light, norepinephrine levels drop, as does synthesis of melatonin. The pineal gland (like the SCN) becomes slightly smaller in summer than in winter, showing how closely tuned our brain is to the seasonal variations we experience in temperate climates.

If any parts of a body's clocklike mechanism are destroyed, the animal or person loses the innate ability to adjust its chronobiological rhythms. The body then becomes out of sync with its surroundings.

To make understanding the phenomenon even more complicated, researchers have discovered that, just as vitamin D stimulates a wide range of cellular functions besides bone mineralization, circadian rhythms are also found at work in many cells of the body outside of the hypothalamus and the brain. They help synchronize the entire body, keeping systems working in harmony with the environment, adjusting sleep, alertness, digestion, mood, immune function, fertility, and more.[3]

In the animal world, the circadian system helps survival by adjusting to successive dawns and dusks. Diurnal animals need to be alert the moment the sun comes up, as predators are all around. It is the same for nocturnal animals who need to be at their sharpest during darkness. Sleep is essential for survival, but it has to come at the proper time. Humans are diurnal—we are up and about in daylight, but barely able to see in the dark. With technology, we have been able to change our limitations. Electric lighting allows us to function even though we are sometimes in a drowsy, fatigued state. Fortunately, we don't have to be at peak performance during all our waking moments as animals in the wild do. In addition to altering our own response to the twenty-four-hour sun cycle, we have also altered the lives of animals reared indoors, such as chickens, dogs, cats, and some commercial livestock and zoo animals.

Candles, lamps, and electricity give us control over our chronobiological systems, allowing us to determine the length of our day and night. But what happens when the natural rhythms of day and night are interrupted? In the short term, we experience fatigue, disorientation, and insomnia. As if enduring a continual case of jet lag, that phenomenon familiar to global travelers, we endure sleepless nights and drag through the day at work. Rotating-shift work pushes people onto longer-term roller-coaster sleep and wake schedules as they are continually readjusting to light and darkness at different points in their workday. When natural rhythms are disturbed, other metabolic systems are pushed out of sync, too, such as the digestive system, kidney function, and hormone levels.

The brain receives messages about light intensity from photoreceptors in the retina via the hypothalamus, which in turn alerts the rest of the brain and the body to the current level of light. Yet some blind people have circadian responses, signaled by eyes that are sightless to form but continue to register light intensity with the hypothalamus. These light signals synchronize the body for sleep, passing the message that light is dwindling and the body can begin shutting down. Upon waking in the morning, different systems are signaled that it is light and time to be on full alert. For this reason, the intact eye is now preserved in people who suffer from certain forms of eye disease that lead to blindness, so the eye can continue its circadian function, although sightless.[4]

These intricate rhythms are interrupted when extended hours of wakefulness at night with bright lights trick our system into adjusting to the light by suppressing melatonin release. If you work late at night under bright artificial lights, your body will not make adequate melatonin during the night while you are sleeping—if you can get to sleep. You've short-circuited the system, or at least unbalanced things, and your body needs to adjust. We've changed our natural daily cycle by extending our day and concentrating our sleep cycle into a shorter period of time and for some people, the disrupted sleep cycle causes problems.[5]

JOHN OTT: PHOTOBIOLOGY PIONEER

John Ott, a photographer, became fascinated by human responses to light when he created innovative time-lapse photography for Walt Disney's films in the 1960s. Ott's "dancing primroses," made by combining a series of photographs of flowers' responses to light combined with waltz music, caught the public's imagination. In order to create photographic sequences of plant growth he had to create innovative studio settings with controlled ultraviolet lighting. He learned how to use lights to get plants to move through natural cycles so he could photograph them continuously in his basement greenhouse-darkroom. As he maneuvered lighting to get plants to move in different directions, he experimented with various types of lighting, gaining an understanding of the ultraviolet spectrum and plant responses to sunlight filtered through glass and plastic coverings.

A few projects he did on animals intrigued him because ultraviolet light had strange and powerful effects on the creatures. During one project in which he was helping a teacher hatch fish eggs, it was revealed that when the light was passed through a pink filter, all the hatchings were female. When the filter was removed they remained female except for about 20 percent that began to show male coloration, but their male secondary sexual characteristics were underdeveloped.[6]

Ott eventually recognized the way ultraviolet light affected his own body when he abandoned first sunglasses, then eyeglasses completely, to obtain unfiltered UV rays from natural sunlight. His eyesight improved when he quit wearing eyeglasses and sunglasses while outdoors working in his yard. During this "experiment" on himself he cut down the amount of time spent under artificial lights indoors and avoided glare, such as that experienced when watching television. He was able to quit wearing eyeglasses, except for reading, and attributed it to the action of natural sunlight on the retina.

Ott's experience is anecdotal, and it may have been due to the increased amount of vitamin D he was getting, too, because he spent several hours a day outdoors in Florida. But Ott strongly believed that because body chemistry is affected by light, the filtering of light to the retina by sunglasses and eyeglass lenses with UV-protective coatings may affect body chemistry and general health.[7]

Ott's work with ultraviolet light, both natural and artificial, is fascinating because he chronicled on film how cells respond to various spectrums of light. His book *Health and Light* is a fascinating must read for anyone interested in learning more about photobiology.[8]

Is it safe to expose the eye to ultraviolet radiation from the sun? While some devotees of "sungazing" claim they receive health benefits from staring at the morning sun, it's dangerous to the delicate structure of the eyeball. According to the Environmental Protection Agency, ultraviolet radiation can increase the likelihood of getting cataracts on the lens of the eye. Other kinds of eye damage include pterygium (tissue growth that can block vision), skin cancer around the eyes, and degeneration of the macula (the part of the retina where visual perception is most acute). All of these problems can be lessened with proper eye protection, such as hats or sunglasses, when in bright sunlight or glare.[9]

RESETTING THE CLOCK

We spend most of our time under incandescent or fluorescent lights, in windowless rooms and cubbies where outdoor light is considered a distraction. Our alarm clocks—rather than the rising sun—wake us and help us adjust to our artificially lighted environment. We work and live indoors, in a continual twilight, where artificial lighting creates a perpetual dusk, compared to natural illumination. While we've been able to reach soaring productivity rates and work anytime we choose, day or night, some of us pay a price for our artificial environment by gaining too much weight, battling seasonal depression, and suffering multiple headaches. Our bodies (and minds) simply cannot function optimally in a continual low-light mode.

Obesity, a current health crisis in temperate climates, has been influenced by calcium and vitamin D levels, as noted in chapters 4 and 5, but it is also linked to chronobiological rhythms. Metabolism changes as autumn and shorter days approach, and the body responds by craving carbohydrates and fats and putting on weight. As if we were preparing for a winter's hibernation, when food stores would be less available, our fat stores begin plumping as the days shorten. Studies done on weight gain between two groups of people on the same diet showed a clear rise in weight gain for the group that received no UV exposure. It helps explain why we put on pounds in winter even while eating the same amount of food as in summer.[10]

Leptin, a hormone found in fat cells, has come under closer scrutiny in recent years. Leptin acts as a satiety factor in regulating food intake and hunger. It controls appetite, signaling either satiation or hunger. A drop in leptin signals the hypothalamus to increase appetite, decrease energy expenditure, and modify neuroendocrine functions in an effort to maintain survival in the face of starvation. As if it were preparing the body for survival mode, falling leptin levels also signal the body to suppress reproduction and activate stress mechanisms.[11] It's not clear, but the amount of leptin in the bloodstream must be fine-tuned—too little or too much and it causes free-running appetite, similar to free-running sleep disorders. Our body's appetite is driven by light; the digestive system responds to melatonin production during the night by shutting down, and serotonin levels in the day turn it back on. Studies are looking at how leptin levels affect appetite and weight gain, as well as what exactly controls leptin levels, which are decidedly linked to photoperiod cycles. Leptin-deficient laboratory mice are obese, diabetic, and sterile, all health problems of increasing importance for many people, too.[12]

Leptin levels in the blood are highest between midnight and 2 AM, and lowest between noon and midafternoon. The similarity with melatonin is strong, suggesting some sort of interaction between the two. Some researchers suggest that obesity may be linked to the production of leptin because young women who gained more weight produced less leptin during the night, which may have been insufficient to quell their appetite during the day. If nighttime levels of leptin are inadequate over a long period of time, it could contribute to the development of obesity by failing to periodically suppress the appetite. Leptin signals the switch from the "fed" to the "starved" state, so a fall in leptin tells the hypothalamus to increase a person's appetite and decrease the individual's energy expenditure—a way to survive when the body faces starvation. When hunger is strong enough, the body finds ways to store energy as fat. Knowledge of how leptin affects the hypothalamus, thyroid, and pituitary may shed more light on obesity.[13]

DAYLIGHT SAVING TIME

Daylight Saving Time (DST) seems an unusual public health topic, but it bears closer scrutiny because it may be affecting the lives of significant numbers of people. DST was a contentious issue when it first surfaced in 1918. It was repealed the following year but reinstituted at state levels, then nationally in the Uniform Time Act of 1966. The law doesn't require all states to participate in adjusting their clocks semiannually, though, and Hawaii, Arizona, and parts of Indiana don't do so. They remain on standard time all year long. Hawaii's daylight hours seldom vary because it's in the tropics, and Indiana residents struggle because the border between Eastern and Central time zones runs through the state, making neighboring towns two hours apart in time. In 2006, all of Indiana adopted DST, but part of the state remains on Eastern Time and part on Central Time. In 2007, DST extended another four to five weeks longer across the entire nation, beginning with the second Sunday in March and extending to the first Sunday of November, due to the Energy Policy Act of 2005.

Establishing clock time and adjusting it to the changing sun have manipulated people's behavior. The sun hasn't changed, it's just that midday (when sun is directly overhead) is 1 PM rather than noon in DST. In Russia, which stretches across eleven time zones, clocks are set one hour ahead of standard time during winter and are moved ahead one more hour in summer. Such a policy has been considered in Britain, too, because it would extend afternoon hours and save fuel. People would be getting up in darkness but having longer afternoons, when it is warmer, and theoretically could save heating energy. No matter how much adjustment we do to our clocks, the earth's revolution is constant—no amount of technology will alter the hours of sunlight. Only moving to a different latitude can do that.[14]

But juggling clocks and watches to try to manipulate sunlight isn't very realistic because it's unnatural and it causes lots of problems. While proponents of DST point to energy savings, there are hidden health costs. The biggest problem seems to be during the period when people are adjusting to slightly different circadian rhythms. The two weeks following either the spring or fall DST time switch is a difficult period for many people.

A shift in what means "morning" and what means "evening," when clocks are readjusted one hour at the very same time the sun is either present or absent for an increasing amount of time, makes it hard to adjust. Nurses working in mental health facilities and adult care centers recognize the influence dusk has on those individuals who are strongly affected by nightfall, becoming restless as evening approaches. When our workday, meals, and usual television programs are altered by an hour, it's hard to know if we are adjusting easily. If our rhythms are adjusted to either morningness or eveningness, how does that affect our work productivity, emotions, and overall functional well-being? For larks, or morning people, who do their best work early in the morning, how are they affected when we shift the time ahead, cutting them short an hour of morning to extend our afternoons in daylight, making the evening later for the owl-type personalities? We don't really know.[15]

DST shows a clear relationship to coordination and judgment. Proponents of DST have held out the fact that having daylight extend into evening hours helps protect pedestrians from drivers who wouldn't see them in the dark. Certainly, that's true. Pedestrian deaths have been found to be lower because DST extended the hours of daylight into early evening. But other studies found that changing time schedules in spring and fall, to DST then back to standard time, led to a significant increase in fatal alcohol-related automobile crashes during the week following both time changes. The increased number of crashes didn't seem to relate to hours of darkness; rather, it may be due to inability to adjust to the sudden switch in chronobiological time. Certainly it's only an hour, but the impact is significant.[16]

Disorders that affect circadian rhythms, such as delayed sleep, interfere with quality of life, such as educational achievement, interpersonal relationships, employment, and personal safety. They affect healthcare costs because fatigue lowers resistance to disease and affects general health status, too. When clock time is artificially altered, on top of a continually changing natural light-dark pattern, our finely tuned circadian rhythms get out of whack. Add to this a rotating night-shift work schedule, and it's a wonder many of us function at all during the natural shifts in seasonal daylight without considering the additional impact of DST.

CLUSTER HEADACHES

Clear connections can be made between circadian rhythm and cluster headaches. Long attributed to a vascular disorder, new findings show that cluster headaches occur in a unique circadian and seasonal pattern. Cluster headaches tend to occur at the same time of year and at the same time of day, nearly clocklike in regularity. The connection to circadian rhythms suggests that our biological clock in the hypothalamus is somehow involved.

According to the International Headache Society, a cluster headache fits a particular definition. To be considered a cluster headache, there should be at least five attacks that fit the following: severe pain across the eyes, above the eyes, or along the temple, lasting 15 minutes to 180 minutes untreated. It's accompanied by at least one of the following on the same side of the head as the headache pain: tears, nasal congestion, runny nose, forehead and facial sweating, constricted pupils, droopy eyelids, or swollen eyelids. The headaches can occur once every other day up to eight times a day. Research on the link between chronobiology and cluster headaches was done two decades ago yet has received little attention. In fact, cluster headaches are often mistaken for seasonal allergies because they occur in fall and spring, close to the equinox.[17]

SEASONAL AFFECTIVE DISORDER

For many, winter means Seasonal Affective Disorder (SAD), a periodic state of depression that begins in autumn and persists until the longer, brighter days of spring. SAD is estimated to affect as many as ten million people, 70 to 80 percent of them women. SAD typically affects people living in the northern latitudes between the months of October and April. SAD sufferers respond naturally to the sun's lower place on the horizon and go into a sort of hibernation. SAD differs from other sorts of depression and seems to be related to preparing our bodies to slow down: it generates carbohydrate craving, weight gain, sluggishness, and sleepiness. SAD sufferers have low energy levels and can become irritable. If these symptoms sound familiar, and you experience them seasonally—meaning they begin in fall and last till spring, then seem to go away with the bright days of summer—perhaps you should see a physician for advice.

SAD is common in northern states but less likely in places like Phoenix or Honolulu. It's a condition directly related to the body's need for sunlight in order to function optimally. If untreated, SAD can affect one's family, job, productivity, and can even be deadly, leading to suicide.

Some effective treatments for SAD include supplementing with doses of vitamin D and using light box therapy. Doses of 400 IU to 800 IU of vitamin D (cholecalciferol) taken daily have reduced depression when given in winter to SAD sufferers.[17] Artificial ultraviolet light therapy, which simulates daylight, was also found to be helpful, especially if begun early in winter and continued until early spring. Therapeutic light boxes are designed to simulate daylight on a cloudy day, at around 2,500 lux. (Lux is a measure of illumination over an area, rather than lumens emitted from a light source. Full sunlight ranges more than 30,000 lux, while average living room lighting is usually about 50 lux.) Exposure for about forty-five minutes, between the hours of 3:30 and 8:00 AM, has shown the best results. The light box works by sending messages about the light to the retina and on to the brain. Early morning light exposure is crucial to resetting the brain's circadian rhythm each day, so a brief session in front of a light box after awakening will make the body think it's morning, even if the exposure occurs at midnight.

SAD can be exacerbated by an erratic sleep schedule, such as that caused by rotating shift work. Interventions to help shift workers adjust to night work and day sleep include wearing dark sunglasses when going outside during the day and while driving home from work, and working under very bright lights during the night shift. Accommodations aren't always effective, however, because it's an attempt to alter an intricately connected system that affects the functioning of several body systems. Researchers still don't completely understand the circadian system, how it works, and how to readjust it. Studying the way serotonin and melatonin work in the body has offered some clues.[18]

Some cases of SAD aren't really seasonal, but appear to happen each day when the sun goes down. Called "Hesperian syndrome," after Hesperia, the Greek goddess of dusk, people who suffer from SAD also sometimes have a reaction to sundown, feeling a looming sadness and a loss of energy.[19]

Surprisingly, SAD shows up more often in young people. Many children and teens have great difficulty getting up early during winter, while in summertime they seem to be up at dawn and full of energy until a late bedtime. Ironically, as autumn settles in, school begins, and kids are forced to be up early and performing well, despite their bodies telling them to slow down and sleep in. During adolescence, the release of melatonin can be disrupted, occurring much later in the night than in adults or children. Whether it's related to hormonal changes of puberty or teens' late-night activities, they don't get sleepy, stay awake until late in the evening, and are unable to get to sleep until far too late to get adequate rest before early morning school start times. They are also not getting adequate sleep time for their bodies to create sufficient amounts of melatonin. Most teens in North America don't get enough sleep in the first place due to evening activities—most involving brightly lit screens—so adding shifting seasonal messages to their circadian system only compounds the difficulty children have adjusting to the length of the day. As the body and melatonin levels struggle to adjust, sleep disorders and associated health problems eventually emerge.

Light box therapy, which provides small amounts of vitamin D as well as exposure to bright lights, has been a popular and often successful treatment for symptoms of SAD, but an alternative solution comes from a new therapy called "dawn simulation." David Avery at Harborview Medical Center in Seattle has been researching dawn simulation using a timed light that brightens to wake one up in the morning. Casting a rosy glow around the bedroom, it wakes you up gradually and naturally, like sunrise. Avery and his colleagues tested three treatment protocols on SAD patients. In one, patients received bright light therapy at 10,000 lux for half an hour, from 6:00 to 6:30 AM. A second group received dawn simulation therapy from a dim light that increased to 250 lux over a ninety-minute time span, from 4:30 to 6:00 AM. A control group received a dim red light (0.5 lux) for ninety minutes from 4:30 to 6:00 AM. After six weeks, those treated with dawn simulation (the second protocol) showed greater remission of SAD symptoms compared to the others.[20]

Dawn simulation works better than light box therapy for many SAD sufferers because it readjusts circadian rhythms to better match the way nature programmed us to respond to sunup, sundown, and long dark winters. Dawn simulation therapy helps adjust sleep patterns and hormone levels and improves mood. But while medical doctors and psychiatrists recommend it, the treatment is not covered by most third-party insurance programs. Medical insurance and public health programs reimburse for pharmaceuticals, but not light therapy equipment.

Vitamin D supplements during the winter may be helpful in alleviating depression symptoms for SAD sufferers.[21] Because low vitamin D levels occur coincidentally during winter when SAD appears, the two seem to be linked. In one small study, SAD patients were given 100,000 IU of vitamin D (cholecalciferol), then compared to a group given only light therapy. After a month, their blood levels were tested for vitamin D; the subjects who were given the large dose of vitamin D showed improvement in all SAD symptoms. Those treated with only light therapy showed a rise in their vitamin D level (made by their skin from the ultraviolet light), but not enough to show any changes in their depression scale scores.

Depression is a disabling condition. Without treatment, SAD can impact every aspect of a person's life, including worker productivity. SAD can affect a region's economy, disabling the work force for long periods of time. Perhaps northern communities and colleges can find ways to supplement the lack of sunshine in winter by providing light therapy to individuals who need it, ensuring a healthier and more productive community.

MELATONIN AND HEALTH

Taking supplemental melatonin is another alternative therapy, which is both popular and controversial. In the 1960s, Julius Axelrod, a biochemist working at the National Institutes of Health, discovered that melatonin is a converted form of serotonin, which the brain's pineal gland regulates to drive the body's circadian rhythm. He laid the foundations for understanding how serotonin and melatonin work to regulate circadian rhythms in the body and won a Nobel Prize for his work. Melatonin is important in sexual maturity, infertility, immune function, and managing lymph organs. Recent findings show it is also an efficient free radical scavenger—an antioxidant—with clinical therapeutic potential in treatments against cell damage resulting from cancers, pulmonary diseases, and neurodegenerative diseases such as Alzheimer's disease. Researchers in Malaysia found melatonin stopped breast cancer cells from multiplying in laboratory studies and inhibited tumor growth of prostate cancer cells in animals. It also helped the body better endure the effects of cancer chemotherapy. It appears to act by stimulating and strengthening the immune system. Those researchers termed it "a natural restraint" on tumor growth. Melatonin has also been found to minimize the effects of aging (at least in laboratory mice).[22]

Melatonin is a naturally occurring hormone made in the brain during the night while one sleeps. As daylight arrives, production of melatonin slows down, eventually shutting off during the day. Essentially, one of the (many) reasons to sleep is so the body can release melatonin—something it cannot do while awake. As melatonin release slows down, other systems begin making serotonin, sending it out to alert the body to perk up for the day. In the United States, melatonin is classified as a food supplement and sold without prescription. Recently it has become popular as an over-the-counter sleep aid. Advocates claim it is useful in correcting insomnia (one of the reactions to mixed-up circadian rhythms). Research needs to be done, but, as Russell Foster and Leon Kreitzman explain in their book, *Rhythms of Life: The Biological Clocks That Control the Daily Lives of Every Living Thing*, because melatonin is a natural substance, commercial interests can't patent it and aren't interested in doing intensive research trials on it. Instead of solid research on melatonin supplementation, they point out, "there is a great uncontrolled trial by the millions who take it." Terry Klassen at the University of Alberta, who authored a review study of melatonin's effect on sleep for the National Institutes of Health's Center for Complementary and Alternative Medicine, echoes that opinion. Large long-term, evidence-based studies to back up popular claims are nonexistent, Klassen points out.[23]

Melatonin has many advocates who self-medicate for a variety of reasons with over-the-counter supplements, often to ameliorate the effects of a sleepless, overstressed lifestyle. Popular with travelers, students studying for exams, and night-shift workers, it's effects are varied. Taking doses of melatonin during the daytime can make you groggy and unfocused, even sleepy. If you're trying to sleep in the daytime, it may relax you so you dose off, but when it's time to be wide awake, your brain won't have received the surge of serotonin it needs. Still, melatonin does seem to help somewhat in adjusting circadian rhythms. Many people find melatonin useful in adjusting to jet lag while traveling on long airplane trips, but the long-term effects of taking it aren't known—there may not be a true advantage and it may create as-yet-unrecognized problems. Taking supplemental melatonin at the same time each day can recalibrate the circadian clock to wake and sleep in a different pattern. At least in research trials it worked with lab mice; but mice are naturally nocturnal, so the results may not be transferable to humans.

While most concern is directed at insomnia or getting enough sleep to function optimally at unnatural times of day, too much sleep can be a problem, too. Sleeping late in the morning allows for too much REM (rapid eye movement) sleep, which has been linked to an increased risk of developing depression. Studies have shown that depression can be linked to the time of waking, with a lower incidence of depression among those who get up before sunrise. Getting up earlier may be helpful for people who suffer from depression; in fact, researchers found that an entire city's rate of depression could be reduced by public health measures to change the time of sunrise—similar to changing Daylight Saving Time year-round. That would change the time on the clock, not the sun of course, so you might simply get up at 6:00 AM, rather than 7:00 AM, but have a half hour before sunrise—time to adjust to the coming dawn. What researchers didn't consider was the reality that most people who are early risers also go to bed earlier in the evening, which may be a significant sign of depression, too.[24]

FERTILITY FINDINGS

Circadian rhythms involve our body's response to changes from light to darkness, a realm that offers potential for greater research, particularly for endocrinology's emphasis on hormones. New studies indicate the light/darkness relationship has a role to play in human fertility, as findings show women undergoing in-vitro fertilization (IVF) treatments have a greater chance of becoming pregnant during the summer months, when levels of sunlight are greatest. For years, it's been known that women are more likely to become pregnant naturally during periods of longer daylight, something we share with many animal species. In 2005, a series of tests in British clinics revealed that between May and September, months when sunlight is most available, women undergoing IVF treatment required significantly lower doses of gonadotrophins (hormones) to stimulate the ovary to produce eggs. Implantation and successful pregnancy rates also increased—in fact doubled—when there was more daily sunlight, with a 15.7 percent success rate compared to 7.5 percent in winter months. Simon Wood at the Countess of Chester Hospital said that melatonin may be the reason "until recently it was thought that melatonin acted only through the pituitary gland in the brain. This natural system is purposefully switched off in women who are undergoing fertility treatment, so it seems that melatonin acts directly on the tissues of the female reproductive system to make it more fertile in lighter months."[25]

ARTIFICIAL LIGHT AND CANCER

While understanding our body's relationship to light and darkness is a challenge, our adoption of artificial lighting to extend working (and waking) hours might also be stimulating cancer tumor growth. In 2005, a research study published in the scientific journal *Cancer Research* found that nighttime exposure to artificial light stimulated the growth of human breast tumors by suppressing melatonin levels. They also found that extended periods of nighttime darkness slowed the growth of breast cancer tumors significantly.

This link between hormonal action and artificially lighted nighttime activity may explain why breast cancer rates are five times higher in industrialized countries than in less-developed areas of the world, and higher in latitudes that experience more seasonal darkness. The increased use of artificial lighting at night in both workplace and home situations suppresses the brain's production of melatonin, the hormone that regulates sleep/wake cycles.

Researchers tested blood samples from the participants (premenopausal women) at three points: after two hours of complete darkness, after ninety minutes of exposure to fluorescent light, and in daylight. The blood samples were then applied to cancer tumors in the laboratory, where they found the blood taken after complete darkness contained melatonin, which severely slowed the growth of the tumors. "The results are due to a direct effect of the melatonin on the cancer cells. The melatonin is clearly suppressing tumor development and growth," said David Blask, lead author on the study. Blood sampled after exposure to fluorescent lighting or daylight, however, stimulated vigorous tumor growth in the lab. A related study published in 2008 found similar cancer rates among postmenopausal women. It appears that low melatonin levels are linked to increased rates of breast cancer for women of all ages.[26] Evidently, the risk of developing breast cancer due to low melatonin levels can be tied to exposure to artificial light at night, independent of female hormonal status.

Working the late shift is understandably problematic for general health, but any activity that continues during evening hours lit by incandescent lighting can be harmful. Women staying up late, trying to get chores accomplished when everyone else is in bed, or even reading for pleasure during the quiet hours, are seriously endangering their health by lowering their melatonin levels. Night-owl lifestyles may take years off our lives. Maybe old Ben Franklin was right about "early to bed, early to rise," even back when candlelight kept people up into the wee hours. "If the link between light exposure and cancer risk can be confirmed, it could have an immediate impact on the production and use of artificial lighting in this country," Richard Stevens, an epidemiologist at the University of Connecticut Health Center, told the NIH.[27]

More recently, scientists are questioning whether it's the lack of darkness at night or the lack of brightness during the day that has the most influence on the development of cancer among people who work night shifts. While the light-at-night hypothesis has been explored in more studies, it appears that the bright-day environment is important when compared to a dim-day environment. Lack of exposure to bright daytime lighting, whether natural or from artificial lighting, may be more important—or at least as important—as whether a person practices staying up late at night in an artificially lighted environment. Richard Stevens notes that perhaps "exposure to a bright day and a dark night, may be a worthy goal." He points out that dosing with pharmacological melatonin supplements in order to remain healthy while working the night shift may have drawbacks. Melatonin supplements given during the daytime, in order to help daytime sleepers get to sleep, may be doing more harm than good because the circadian rhythm based on darkness and light is also essential. Supplementation at the wrong time of day (in daytime, rather than just before bedtime) may flood the body with melatonin at the wrong time of day, confusing the system and creating "circadian disruption." The exposure to light at night, at first considered to be the cause of cancer because it disrupted melatonin creation, which allowed estrogen levels to increase, may be only part of the story. Exposure to bright daytime lighting appears to play a stronger role in whether the body creates much melatonin later during sleep at night. Our dim daytimes, with low-level office and home lighting, along with wearing sunglasses when going outdoors, may be keeping us at a daytime level too low for optimal health.[28]

While this book is about sunlight, it's opposite, darkness, appears to be important to our health as well. As researchers at the University of Texas Health Science Center noted in 2007, "It is apparent that true darkness is disappearing. For years it was assumed that polluting the daily dark period with light was inconsequential in terms of animal/human physiology." They feel that is incorrect, because "light at night has two major physiological actions: it disrupts circadian rhythms and suppresses the production of melatonin by the pineal gland." That is crucial, because epidemiological studies now show some relationship between night work and the development of breast, prostate, endometrial, and colorectal cancers. In laboratory animals, results of exposing animals to light at night or shifting their chronobiological clocks with lighting show a higher cancer risk. And, as they point out, we're only looking at the effect of lighting on cancer tumors; there may be many other diseases affected by artificial lighting suppressing the body's creation of melatonin at night.[29]

It's clear that without enough ultraviolet radiation from sunshine, followed by regular periods of darkness, health suffers. Without adequate exposure to natural daylight and rhythmic light-dark cycling, performance and behavior also suffer. While seasonal affective disorder (SAD) leads to depression, weight gain, and fatigue for many during winter months, daily sunlight exposure is as important as seasonality. Yet most of us are stuck in classrooms, workplaces, or homes, under electric lights all day long and into the night. Getting outdoors as much as possible is crucial, but indoor access to daylight can also improve our situation.

DAYLIGHTING INDOORS

"Daylighting" in buildings—providing natural light through windows or sky-lights—provides high-quality illumination during the day while saving electricity and air conditioning costs. Before the 1940s, most buildings used daylight as the primary light source. Twenty years later, virtually all indoor illumination was artificial.

There are four basic types of lightbulbs used indoors; each uses a different portion of the light spectrum:

- Cool white fluorescent uses the yellow to red end of the spectrum
- Incandescent lights use the orange to red end of the spectrum
- Energy-efficient fluorescent uses the yellow to green portion of the spectrum
- Full-spectrum fluorescent uses the yellow to blue end and is the only artificial light to include a blue portion of the spectrum

The blue portion of the light spectrum is the most important for humans and is best provided by natural light. Natural daylight peaks slightly in the blue-green area of the spectrum.[30]

Low-light indoor environments, created by low-lux or partial spectrum lighting, can affect our internal circadian rhythms because the brain never gets a signal that it is bright enough to shut off melatonin production. As a result, we get that groggy, depressed feeling during the day. The body is working in a continual dusk, trying to turn on sleep mechanisms while we're at work or school. Meanwhile workers in buildings lit by daylight or full-spectrum bulbs enjoy an increased general sense of well-being, as well as increased energy and productivity. Benefits are so important that many countries in Europe now require workers to be positioned within twenty-seven feet of a window.[31]

When windows are impossible, full-spectrum bright lights help keep workers alert by signaling their internal circadian cycles to stop producing melatonin. Exposure to natural lighting helps avoid the common after-lunch dip in energy levels many people feel.

In today's work environment, windows still go to the higher-status employees. The corner office with a window has long been coveted as the ultimate workplace perk, the window more sought after than the privacy. Companies that modified the workspace to gain more windows, such as Lockheed Martin (up by 15 percent), VeriFone (25 to 28 percent), and West Bend (16 percent), found substantial increases in worker productivity. In several instances, worker absenteeism shrank between 15 and 25 percent when daylight was added to buildings.[32]

It's hard to overcome ingrained beliefs that windows in classrooms distract students and that the benefits of windowless schoolrooms (more bulletin board space, heating efficiency, security) are outweighed by the advantages of natural daylight. Building design, including inner atriums, skylights, and mirrors, can make a difference for students and teachers.

Classrooms without windows are very stressful places for children and adolescents. Students in windowless classrooms are more hostile, hesitant, maladjusted, unmotivated, and apt to complain. Studies show that children in daylit classrooms enjoy improved eyesight, increased growth, and better immune systems.

Daylighting can also be an effective way to prevent tooth decay. There are several studies linking kids' dental decay to school lighting. Cavities were reduced when daylight or full-spectrum bulbs were used in classrooms. In one study, tooth decay decreased by nine times. Hamster experiments found those reared under cool-white fluorescent lights had five times the tooth decay as those reared under full-spectrum fluorescents. The link between vitamin D and calcium metabolism appears to play a part.[33]

Achievement, too, is affected by classroom lighting. In Johnston County, North Carolina, students in daylit schools scored higher on reading and math achievement tests than their counterparts in artificially lighted schools. One school in the county was destroyed by fire then rebuilt while students moved to artificially lit rooms. Test scores before the fire, during the interim, and in a new windowed building were compared. Before the fire, students placed 7 percent above the county average on the California Achievement Test. During the two years they spent in windowless rooms, test scores fell to 10 percent below the average. In the new building with natural lighting, scores moved up to 9 percent above average the first year. Impressed by those results, the county built two more elementary schools with daylighting design and saw average test scores rise by 7 and 18 percent, respectively.[34]

Comparisons between students in the same school but with different room lighting showed higher scores for students exposed to the most daylight. In Orange County, California, students with more daylight became 20 percent faster in learning math and 26 percent faster in reading. In Seattle, students with more daylight had 9 percent higher math scores and 13 percent higher reading scores than counterparts in artificially lit rooms. In Fort Collins, Colorado, scores averaged 7 percent higher in both reading and math for students with more daylight.[35] So for communities interested in increasing students' test scores, adding windows may be one of the most sensible and rewarding educational reforms.

Other studies show that full-spectrum fluorescent lighting, which replicates daylighting, calmed hyperactive students and generated overall better behavior in students than fluorescent-lit schools. Many districts are moving ahead, incorporating daylight into new buildings to improve performance. In 2001, Connecticut legislated that construction or renovation of schools must maximize natural light or use full-spectrum fluorescent lighting.[36]

Retail stores are at the forefront of daylighting design because people want to be in spaces that are aglow with natural light. Customers feel more positive and upbeat inside naturally lit stores, and they want to spend more time (and money) there. The nation's largest chain retailers have opted for plenty of windows, and new shopping centers feature skylights and atriums, creating a feeling that the buildings are cleaner, brighter, and more spacious to shoppers. Consultants estimate that adding skylights to a non-daylit store improves store performance by 31 to 49 percent—significantly paying back the investment.[37]

Substantial research supports the use of daylight in nursing homes, hospitals, schools, and the workplace. In building design, emphasis should be placed on maximizing daylight as much as construction and maintenance costs. Natural light can make us healthier, happier, and more productive. Like houseplants, we too, need windows, greenhouses, atriums, or full-spectrum lights.

In the end, there's nothing that can take the place of natural sunlight when it comes to optimum health. Our circadian and biological rhythms are essential to a host of physical functions: digestion, body temperature, kidney cycles, hormones, immunity to disease, cognition, motor coordination, and mood. Over a millennia, we've adapted to living at latitudes that challenge our bodies due to fluctuating levels of sunlight. Today, however, we exacerbate the difficulty by keeping ourselves in the shadows much of the time and under artificial lighting. We've compounded the problems our internal clocks face by working late, sleeping at noon, and wearing sunglasses or staying indoors all the time.

But there are ways to supplement our lack of sunlight and the cost is not very high. Light box therapy, dawn simulators, as well as full-spectrum lights at home, school, and work, are all easy to incorporate into daily life. With huge savings in increased worker productivity, better school performance, and decreased healthcare costs, perhaps resetting clocks and watches is the easiest way to bring more of the crucial morning sunlight into our lives. Other issues, such as eliminating rotating work shifts, need more attention. Of all the remedies, it's the one that hits the bottom line; the only adjustment that really costs much money. We long ago abandoned the ideal of the "city on a hill" for a modern, industrial "city that never sleeps." Many are paying the price, with insomnia, fatigue, and depression.

Maybe it's time for everyone to turn out the lights and get a good night's sleep.

Chapter Eight

SOLAR DIMMING AND HEALTH

The world is becoming a darker place, not just because we've moved indoors, but because the sun's radiation is no longer as strong as it once was. Since the 1950s, sunlight dimming has reduced the amount of sunlight reaching the earth's surface by as much as 10 to 37 percent. The amount of sunshine we are getting is dropping by 2 to 3 percent a decade. In Asia, the United States, and Europe, at northern latitudes, the amount has decreased up to 37 percent since the late 1950s.[1]

Global dimming, as the phenomenon is called, is a recent discovery. Before 2001, few scientists had heard of the topic or even realized that sunlight was diminishing. The data reveal that between the 1950s and 1990, the amount of sunlight reaching the ground had dropped by 9 percent in Antarctica, 10 percent in the United States, 30 percent in Russia, 22 percent in Israel, and 16 percent in the British Isles. One recent study found that the dimming may have slowed in the 1990s over the Northern Hemisphere and the amount of sunlight actually increased, suggesting that the skies have become slightly clearer. There may be some slight clearing over areas where general air pollution has reduced, such as Germany, but it's too early to tell if the dimming trend has slowed.[2]

What caused the dimming? Experts suspect it's due to air pollution. Tiny particles circle the earth, reflecting the sun's rays back away from the earth's surface. The polluting particles are thought to be soot. The floating particles also trap evaporating water, causing more water droplets to condense and form as cloud cover, which also blocks sunlight. Areas of the globe with less air pollution, such as the Southern Hemisphere, haven't experienced as much dimming as others, but even Antarctica is receiving less sunshine. Satellites measuring the sun's radiation record it to be as strong as ever, so the cause isn't that the sun is burning itself out. It's just that less radiation is reaching the ground.

LESS SUNLIGHT SINCE 1950s

Scientists began noticing the dimming about twenty years ago, but unbelievers scoffed at their findings. Radiometers to record sunshine had been set up around the globe in the 1950s in what was believed to be a fairly systematic way to help monitor climate. In the 1980s, a researcher began looking at the data and realized it was impossible to correlate because the amount of sunlight in various places was diminishing. He told a reporter for the *New York Times* that he couldn't believe what he found. Skeptical colleagues rebuked and ignored him. Similar findings by Dr. Gerald Stanhill at Israel's Ministry of Agriculture, which monitored sunlight for decades in order to moderate irrigation water for crops in Israel, supported the dimming theory. In the Bavarian Alps, Beate Liepert, a graduate student in climatology, documented a drop in sunlight in Germany, too. Other researchers, working independently, found that long-term data collection on water evaporation showed there was a diminished amount of sunshine.[3]

But if sunlight has been diminishing so quickly, why haven't we gotten colder? To understand the situation, experts point to the global warming phenomenon. The fact that the earth's surface hasn't been getting warmer has been one of the main tenets of the argument against global warming. Critics claim that since the earth isn't getting warmer—just wetter—there's no significant global warming phenomenon. But with a protective cloud cover due to global dimming, we're not getting the normal amount of sunlight. The pollution overhead is actually insulating us from the heat we would be receiving due to the destruction of the ozone layer, which lies far above the clouds. The destruction of the ozone layer by industrial processes on the ground has opened us up to intense radiation from the sun. Yet, with the protection of pollution-generated cloud cover, the radiation isn't reaching us. The clouds are trapping the carbon dioxide we're emitting, generating wildly erratic weather patterns that include record amounts of precipitation in the form of rainfall and snow. Even fog, a dangerous nuisance to airline pilots and automobile commuters, has been increasing and can be explained by the cloud layer that traps it from above.

EVAPORATION RATE

Global dimming and global warming seem to contradict each other, but research on evaporation helps connect the two. Two Australian biologists, Michael Roderick and Graham Farquahar, noticed a worldwide decline in the "pan evaporation" rate. Namely, that's the rate at which water evaporates out of a pan. Agricultural scientists and others measure the process, keeping track of how much water they must add to the pan to restore the original water level. It's been an innocuous job, going on for the past century. Roderick and Farquahar were puzzled when evaporation rates slowed in the 1990s. They discovered that it isn't heat from the sun that causes water to evaporate, as long believed, but light irradiating the liquid water molecules, causing them to vibrate and evaporate as water vapor. Less light equals slower evaporation rates.[4]

It didn't take them long to calculate evaporation rate declines around the globe that matched the climatologists' findings on sunlight decline. Independent scientists, working on climatology and agriculture, had come up with the same conclusions.

Veerabhadran Ramanathan of the University of California set up tests in the Maldive Islands, an archipelago in the Indian Ocean, to figure out what was causing global dimming. The northern Maldives receive more cloud cover, as they are in-line with pollution spewed from India's industrial zone; the southern Maldives are in a pristine setting with air coming from Antarctica. The study took four years, twenty-five million dollars, and participation from several nations. The work produced results. Ramanathan told an interviewer for the BBC program *Horizon*, "The stunning part of the experiment was [that] this pollutant layer which was three kilometers thick, cut down the sunlight reaching the ocean by more than 10 percent." Particles of soot, sulfates, nitrates, and ash were trapped in clouds, reflecting sunlight away from the earth, thereby capturing more water molecules and causing more rainfall.[5]

Because less solar energy reaches earth's surface, all of the environmental weather patterns we have adjusted our lives around are now out of kilter. More rainfall in one area of the world impacts other areas, too, interrupting natural weather patterns. Clouds act as rainfall sponges, or shields, depending upon the changing temperature of the oceans below. Climatologists now blame the drought of the African Sahel in the 1980s and 1990s on monsoon rain patterns that have dropped 15 percent since the 1980s due to the warming of the Indian Ocean. We have long believed the African drought was due to overgrazing and poor land management, but now it appears the change in weather patterns is the culprit. Scientists predict no end in sight to the central African drought, estimating the lack of rainfall due to oceanic warming to continue.[6]

Ironically, the diminished sunlight is a factor in cooling oceans in some areas while it creates drought in other areas. Around the world, it's been clear to see historic weather records overturned by record rainfall, snow depths, and heat waves in various regions. Tornadoes and hurricanes, which relate to the temperature of the ground and clouds, have become more unpredictable and violent.

EFFECTS ON AGRICULTURE

Now, as we embark on life under a growing cloud cover, researchers are mining the data from the past century, trying to figure out what to expect. Some studies on the effects of cloudy skies on plants are available, and they show interesting results. When plants are in an adequate situation as far as temperature and water go but are reared in shaded conditions (under netting screens), they develop very differently from their normal growth patterns. Much more of a plant's energy goes into leaf and stem growth, with energy being taken away from the root system. Plants develop much larger amounts of "biomass," meaning plant material. Leaves get larger, stems are wider and longer—the whole plant is spreading its tissues out to become as large as possible, trying to absorb more sunlight with a larger surface area. Crop yields are smaller because so much energy has gone into making biomass in an attempt by plants to capture more sunlight for photosynthesis.[7]

This oversized growth by plants is eerily reminiscent of what we know about the age of the dinosaurs. Skies were clouded with pollutants from volcanic eruptions and huge wildfires, and the climate was humid and wet due to the thick layer of cloud cover over the earth—a result of the suspended pollutants in the atmosphere. Plants were huge then; gingko leaves were the size of dinner plates and ferns grew twenty feet tall.

It's just a wild idea, of course, great fodder for arguments about global warming and something many will likely enjoy ridiculing. But while it seems crazy to think that our planet could return to the conditions of the Mesozoic era, our continued burning of coal and petroleum—spewing particles into the air with abandon—means everything has come full circle. It is ironic that we're thickening the skies overhead by burning carbon from plants that desperately sought sunlight for photosynthesis in an earlier, dimly lit epoch.

Sunlight changes affect plants, and that directly affects the world's agricultural stability. A new phenomenon linked to pollutants, "atmospheric brown clouds," or "ABCs," are created by burning fossil fuels, and the biomass blocks sunlight radiation in many parts of the world. By reflecting sunlight back into space, the clouds block the sunlight plants need for photosynthesis and optimal growth. Recent research shows that these dirty clouds reduce rainfall as well, by reducing surface evaporation from the ocean—a process that relies on sunlight.

Researchers in India discovered that rice crops were diminished due to the increased number of ABCs that skewed both rainfall and ultraviolet light available to rice plants. Rice is a sensitive crop, needing adequate rainfall as well as plenty of solar radiation late in the season. As the conditions dried and dimmed, rice crop yields fell between 6 to 17 percent. That reduction in yield can have tremendous impact in areas of Southeast Asia that rely on rice as a mainstay of the food supply.[8]

The Green Revolution, which introduced chemical farming methods to the developing world, created increased yields after the mid-1960s, but those gains leveled off by the early 2000s, and a deceleration has begun. Experts blame a variety of reasons for the downward trend in agricultural productivity, citing deteriorating irrigation systems, overworked land, and low crop prices. Adding to these factors, the decline in solar radiation reaching rice plants as they mature and ripen, along with the lowered annual rainfall, mean many parts of the world are in jeopardy, facing decreasing food supplies. Researchers at the University of California believe that the ABC effect was responsible for more than a 10 percent drop in rice production between 1985 and 1998.[9]

SAVE OUR SUNLIGHT

The carbon-based fuels we use today are from the layers of decayed plants that flourished at a time when the earth was a dim, wet, warm paradise for things like cockroaches and crocodiles. The mammals disappeared. We could encounter a similar fate, because no amount of technology can allow us to live sustainably on a cloud-shrouded earth. We can make a change, however. Scientists point to an urgent need to decrease the burning of coal (we're burning more now than at the height of the industrial age at the turn of the twentieth century, and we're spewing the waste higher into the atmosphere while not letting it waft through the neighborhood), to burn it with more cleaners and scrubbers in place, to cut back on petroleum-based fuels that spew tiny particles into the air. Research is needed to cut back the pollution that hangs overhead, trapping us in clouds. The second phase is to restore the ozone, or at least slow its destruction. It forms a natural protective buffer between the sun and us.

Experts say we can minimize the amount of petroleum fuels we burn by adding scrubbers to power stations, catalytic converters in cars, and using low-sulfur fuels. These practices have cut down on visible air pollution.

We can also turn to locally produced and grown products to minimize the amount of pollution from transportation—there is no need to ship fruits and flowers by air freight. We should rethink nuclear power, creating smaller, safer systems as found in Europe. We should immediately stop practices such as burning logging debris and farm fields after harvest, which adds tons of par-ticulates to the air overhead.

What many now think is that the protective action of global dimming has lulled us into not seeing how at risk we are from global warming. The layer of pollutants and cloud cover has hidden the greenhouse gases that have heated up the atmosphere far more than we previously thought. And no one has men-tioned the need we have for adequate amounts of sunlight in order to create vitamin D. We may want to retreat into our electrically lit buildings, but it's the worst thing we can do for our health.

MICROBIAL DUST

While much concern about global warming has been about how it relates to agriculture, the microbes borne on blowing dust has been overlooked. Drought conditions on one continent affect others because dust blows up into the atmosphere, where it is carried by winds. Dust also comes from burning forests and croplands. The dust clouds are huge (now a billion tons per year from Africa) and have been sweeping out of Africa's desert regions, across the Atlantic Ocean, and depositing African dust over about 30 percent of the North American continent. Florida and the Caribbean receive about half of the total amount carried across the seas. A blanket of dust clouds deflect the sun's radiation in the southern United States, where the more intense dust storm months are June through October, at latitudes up to 25 degrees. The particles are so small that the sky appears clear on the ground below, so it's hard to realize the vast number of ultra-tiny particles that remain in the air. We breathe in the particles, often without recognizing distress. In Florida, during a summertime walk outdoors, 50 percent of the particles residents breathe in come from Africa, four thousand miles away.[10]

In the Pacific, dust clouds move dust from the Gobi Desert great distances, particularly when winds over ocean currents move them quickly. Asian dust is dispersed around the world in the Northern Hemisphere; in 1990, deposits from Asia moved across the Pacific Ocean, over the continent of North America and the Atlantic Ocean, before being dumped on the French Alps. Four thousand tons of dust per hour from Asian deserts can be swept to the Arctic. In 1998, one cloud off the west coast of North America reduced solar radiation levels by 30 to 40 percent and swept dust as far as Minnesota. In Los Angeles, it's estimated that at times one-fourth of the city's smog consists of pollution blown in from China.[11]

Airborne dust from Asia has increased in the last twenty years, attributed to both climate change and desertification. China's environment is degrading rapidly, showing a desertification rate between 1975 and 1987 of 2,100 km^2—about 800 square miles—per year. Those data were gathered years before today's booming Chinese economy, which has been responsible for tons of additional pollutants being poured into the skies. Today, with industrial expansion in full tilt across China, the problem is much worse. As host city to the 2008 Olympic Games, Beijing went on a concerted cleanup effort to eliminate polluted skies from ruining the games. Two million cars were kept off the roads and dirty factories were shut down for weeks before the games began. The effort made the city proud, with extraordinarily clean air at times. Despite the effort, however, pollutants still clouded the skyline because 75 percent of the pollution over Beijing actually blows into the city of 17 million people from outside—dust blown in from the expanding deserts and coal smoke from factories elsewhere. The situation continues to worsen, with pollutants now blown across the Pacific Ocean from China in plumes nearly two miles high, moving up into the jet stream and across the Pacific in three to four days. As in the Sahel of Africa, the pollution adds to the desertification of the region because the pollution clouds actually prevent rainfall in China, intensifying the drought conditions there.[12]

While the dirty dust clouds add to environmental problems by creating extremes in rainfall or drought, it's important to recognize that they may create serious health problems as well, for people, animals, and plants. Dust sweeps up into the atmosphere with a variety of particles: sand and dirt, as well as plant pollens, fungal spores, dried animal feces, minerals, chemicals from fires and industrial plants, and pesticide residue. Until recently, no one considered that the dust also included a wide variety of land-dwelling microbes. Numerous microbes—viruses and bacteria—are carried along with the airborne dust, some attached to the dust itself. Under normal conditions, sunlight sanitizes the dust carried in the air, killing microbes with ultraviolet radiation. A higher layer of fine particles from pollutants and water vapor is now spread across the upper atmosphere, and this layer acts as a shield, reflecting sunlight away from the earth's surface. Dimming ultraviolet radiation, along with the thickness of the blowing dust clouds, means sunshine simply isn't working as well as it should to eliminate microbes and sanitize the dust before it falls to earth.[13]

The huge amount of dust in these plumes means the dust particles shadow the microbes below them, and the sunlight is dimmer than it used to be due to pollutants in the upper atmosphere above the dust cloud. That combination of higher layers of pollutants with a lower cloud of dust limits the sun's ability to sterilize bacteria and viruses as effectively as it once did. It's a concern for the world's health, but particularly for North America, because dust plumes are sweeping onto the continent from both East and West coasts, spreading untold numbers of microbes as the particles settle to the ground or onto waterways. There's a ring of dirty particles high in the atmosphere over North America already. "You can actually see this bathtub ring around the Northern Hemisphere," Stanley A. Morain, head of the Earth Data Analysis Center at the University of New Mexico, points out. That ring acts as sunglasses, reflecting the sun's rays, and ironically, protecting the ground below from the full force of warming.[14]

Dale W. Griffin, a scientist with the US Geological Survey, is researching African and Asian dust clouds because they pose a potential threat to public health. The inability of the sun to sterilize the dust plumes has created a new vehicle for the global transport of pathogens. "It is clear that a very diverse population of microorganisms, including fungi, bacteria, and viruses is moving vast distances in Earth's atmosphere," Griffin explains. "A significant fraction (20 to 30 percent) of this cultivable population (bacteria and fungi) consists of species capable of causing disease in a wide range of organisms (trees, crop plants, and animals)."[15]

Findings show that 20 to 30 percent of the microbes in dust clouds cause disease to animals or people. So far, no devastating epidemic has been linked to the tainted dust, but microbes that cause ear infections, skin lesions, and mouth sores are among the many that have been identified. Human diseases such as coccidioidomycosis (a flulike condition caused by inhaling fungal spores, which can last eight weeks or longer), Al Eskan disease (sometimes called Desert Storm pneumonitis, because it appeared in troops exposed to desert dust storms in the Persian Gulf), and desert lung syndrome (a lung infection found in the desert Southwest) have been carried in dust. Dust deposits tested in Mali, a central African nation that receives dust plumes from the Sahara, are found to carry bacteria responsible for gastrointestinal illnesses, septicemia (blood poisoning), and staphylococcus (bacterial infection that can lead to pneumonia). In the "meningitis belt" of northern Africa, two hundred thousand people a year get meningitis during dust storms.[16]

Could airborne microbes be a larger problem than any other we've experienced with global warming? Certainly airborne microbes have been well studied in agriculture because crops are easily affected by dispersal of airborne fungal pathogens, particularly in field crops like wheat and corn. Dust storms have spread foot-and-mouth disease among livestock in Korea and Japan, following dust storms coming out of the Gobi Desert, where the disease is endemic. In one case, airborne *Acinetobacter calcoaceticus* has been linked to spreading mad cow disease.[17]

"It is tempting to speculate that transatlantic transport of dust could be a vector to renew reservoirs of some plant and animal pathogens in North America and could also be the cause of new diseases," according to Griffin. Foot-and-mouth, meningitis, influenza, and anthrax are a few of the diseases that might affect us this way, but there's potential for many more to appear that we've never experienced. Also, the conditions may make mutations possible, giving us diseases that have never existed before. One gram of desert soil can contain as many as 1 billion bacteria cells, and without the sun's protective cleansing action, we have no idea what the future holds.[18] Studies from the National Aeronautics and Space Administration (NASA) show the dust clouds can diminish ultraviolet sterilization of microbes by more than 50 percent. The speed at which these microbes reach the Americas is astounding: Asian dust storms can travel from the Gobi Desert to the West Coast of North America in seven days, and dust from the coast of Africa reaches the Caribbean and Florida coast in three to five days.[19]

As William A. Sprigg, a University of Arizona climate expert, notes, "We are just beginning to accumulate the evidence of airborne dust implications on human health. Until now, it's been like the tree falling in the forest. Nobody heard, so nobody knew it was there."[20] There is little being done to study the problem, one that most governments would rather ignore. As Eugene Shinn, the scientist who linked a disease affecting coral reefs in the Caribbean to microbes blown in from Africa, explains, "No government agency wants to face this problem because no one knows what to do about it." He warns, "In my opinion nothing will change regarding either African or Asian dust until we have a catastrophe such as a large-scale avian flu, West Nile virus, or some other deadly outbreak that cannot be explained away by the usual suspects." Sprigg, now retired, feels his warnings have been futile in the face of the growing threat of airborne microbes. Government and health officials do not see the larger picture, which in this case is global. "We will continue to employ agents to check for fruit in baggage and dirt on tourists' shoes," he notes, "while hundreds of millions of tons of soil dust carrying live microbes continue to be transported unchecked overhead."[21]

Meanwhile, there is no clear body of research regarding the problem in the field of "aerobiology," nor is there widespread recognition that sunlight's role is so vital to sanitizing the world's air. It will take a combination of new work from a variety of scientific fields to clarify the threats we may be facing. Whether we are struck by powerful pandemics as microbes hit the continent within days, or are weakened insidiously by little-known or mutated microbes, no one has a clear understanding of what's happening at this point. As Dale Griffin, a leading researcher in the field, said, "It is clear that we have only begun to grasp the true numbers of microorganisms capable of using the atmosphere as an infectious route."[22]

Sunlight's importance as the great sanitizing force for the planet, necessary for the health and well-being of all living things, is evident. Getting more sunlight, keeping pollutants out of the atmosphere, and protecting the ozone layer are imperative for everyone's survival. The problems are global in scale, however, and recognizing the situation has been our most difficult hurdle. Now that scientists are putting the pieces of the puzzle together, we may be better equipped to understand and protect our relationship with the sun. Ancient civilizations understood the sun was not a force to be ignored—it is time for us to rethink our relationship with it as well.

EPILOGUE

It's clear that we need light in a variety of ways: for healthy physical processes and avoidance of chronic disease, as well as for mental stability and acuity due to natural shifting chronobiological rhythms. Recognizing our need for sunlight and how much is optimal is only the tip of the iceberg, however, because implementing more sunlight and vitamin D into our lives will mean adjusting our lifestyles. It means we'll have to venture outdoors into natural light as often as possible, perhaps even so drastic as shifting our view of work and its value. Indoor work done with computer screens and keyboards might become a less desirable form of labor, while mowing lawns or being a playground monitor may become increasingly desirable. However we shift ourselves to embrace the light, as we do so, our lives will change considerably from the indoor, sheltered focus we've created in the past century.

As we move outdoors more, protecting our access to sunlight becomes significant—in fact, crucial. Pollutants filling the skies overhead reflect the solar rays away from us, weakening our health. Sun rights, something not recognized since Roman days when homes were constructed to provide access to solar warmth and brightness, might become a real human rights issue. Particulates from burning coal, smoke from agriculture and forestry, and clouds of humidity brought about through the warming of the seas will all endanger our access to the sun's healing rays. Protecting our right to sunlight will become a future challenge.

Because living an outdoor life isn't possible for everyone, supplementation with vitamin D is increasingly essential and is needed at higher levels than in the past. Research supports a changing of the guard, so to speak, as medical professionals push the FDA and medical societies to adopt higher levels of vitamin D intake for well-being. A similar example occurred with folic acid in the recent past, with debates raging for decades over the need for increasing recommended levels. Research pointed to a lack of folic acid in most diets, its disappearance from foods produced by industrial agriculture methods, and the strong relationship between deficiency and birth defects. Like vitamin D, folic acid could be harmful in very high amounts (it masks vitamin B_{12} deficiency).

Eventually, opposing groups within the food and medical community came to an understanding, a small amount of folic acid was added to fortify grain products, and pregnant women were advised to take supplements. The increased consumption of folic acid has cut the incidence of neural tube defects in newborns by more than 50 percent.

Vitamin D will likely follow the same contested regulatory pathway. Sadly, many individuals suffer lifelong health consequences as interest groups within the regulatory, medical, and food community battle over minimal issues for years.

Our actions will be mirrored in future generations. Research into the emerging science of epigenetics—how our genes are affected by our environment and passed on to the next generation—is just now touching on vitamin D and how it affects human genetics. Can we survive over time as indoor dwellers? How that affects future generations is relatively unknown. It's likely to be even more important in the future, as microbe-filled clouds of dust, no longer cleansed by the sun's rays, fill our lungs. We'll need to rely on our immune systems to repel the tiny invaders, immune systems that will hopefully not be so compromised by lack of vitamin D that we cannot survive. It's time to remember we are not the center of the universe, but just one planet in one solar system that revolves around the sun.

GLOSSARY

Analog. A drug that differs a bit from the molecular compound it is designed to simulate. It may be more potent or without certain harmful side effects found in the original compound. Calcipotriene is a vitamin D analog, which is sold as the medication Dovonex for the treatment of psoriasis.

Autoimmune disease. Several unrelated diseases now believed to be the result of inflammation and destruction of tissues by the body's own immune system. The body's immune system seems unable to tell the difference between "self" molecules and invasive "other" molecules, and turns on the immune system to destroy what it detects as invaders. It seems to involve defective cells creating antibody protection that attacks the body's own cells.

Basal cell carcinoma. The most common kind of skin cancer. It grows and spreads very slowly. It is most often found on the face of light-skinned people, is usually linked to years of sunlight exposure, and most often occurs with aging. While it is not life-threatening, dermatologists usually cut or freeze the small lesions to remove them.

Beriberi. A vitamin deficiency condition caused by inadequate amounts of thiamine (B_1). Advanced cases can result in death from degeneration of the nervous system and heart failure.

Calcidiol 25(OH)D. Calcidiol is created by the body from cholecalciferol and circulates in the bloodstream. Blood tests for vitamin D usually identify the amount of calcidiol in the bloodstream. Tests for calcidiol measure 25-hydroxyvitamin D levels.

Calcitriol 1,25(OH)2D3 D3. The kidneys turn calcidiol from the bloodstream into calcitriol, a form of steroid hormone. It is the "active" form of vitamin D, which is sent out to cells.

Carcinoma. Cancer occurring in the epithelium, the skin on the body's exterior and on the lining of internal organs. It is a cancer that can occur in any of the epithelial cells, from the skin surface on the face to the lining of the cervix. It refers to the location of the cancer, not the type of tumor.

Cell differentiation. Stem cells are directed by DNA to express certain genes in their daughter cells. Those daughter cells become specialized for assigned functions and are unable to change their destiny. Out of fetal cells, for example, cells will become nerve, muscle, or skin cells. It is sort of a cell's assignment when it is created.

Cell proliferation. An increase in the number of similar cells as cells grow and divide.

Cholecalciferol. Vitamin D_3. This is the naturally occurring form of vitamin D made in the skin when exposed to ultraviolet radiation from the sun or UV lights. It can be absorbed through the digestive system, too, from food sources. Synthetic cholecalciferol is made by exposing wool to UV lights, extracting the resulting cholecalciferol from the fat cells of the wool fibers, and refining it chemically. The extract is dried to a powder form and sold as a dietary supplement or used in food fortification.

Chronobiology. The study of how living organisms adapt to biological rhythms related to the sun and moon, from annual patterns to less-than-daily cycles.

Circadian rhythms. Physiological responses to light and darkness patterns during a twenty-four-hour cycle.

Daylighting. Incorporating natural light into a building through windows or skylights.

Dystocia. Difficult childbirth usually caused by a too-large fetus, inability of the cervix to begin labor, or inadequate pelvic bone structure.

Ergocalciferol. Vitamin D_2, or sometimes just called calciferol. It is a form of vitamin D found in fungi that have been exposed to ultraviolet light or sunlight. When mushrooms are irradiated, the plant ergosterol converts to calciferol, or D_2. It is the form of vitamin D that physicians prescribe, not often used in food fortification. Scientists thought it was not as well absorbed as cholecalciferol, but studies beginning in 1999 found that irradiated mushrooms created significant amounts of calcidiol in the bloodstream.

Ergosterol. A plant sterol that converts to the vitamin D_2 form of ergocalciferol after it has been exposed to ultraviolet radiation from sunlight or artificial light sources.

Fluorescent lights. Used in most commercial buildings, they generate visible light but not much heat. Fluorescent lights can emit the full spectrum of light but usually do not. The most common, the cool-white fluorescent tube, emits very little red or blue-violet light, colors that are most like sunlight. Unless it is "full-spectrum" type, fluorescent bulbs are the least like sunlight of all bulbs.

Full-spectrum lights. Lightbulbs designed to simulate the brilliance of natural outdoor light at noontime. They are not the bulbs sold as "daylight" but are a clear, white light. They were first patented by John Nash Ott.

Hypercalcuria. Excessive calcium in the urine, usually the cause of calcium kidney stone disease.

Hypervitaminosis D. Excess of vitamin D in the body. Can lead to too much calcium in the blood and can produce kidney stones.

Incandescent lights. Ordinary household lightbulbs, which emit mostly yellow and red light, and almost no light in the blue or ultraviolet light spectrum. We use it for visible lighting and as a heat source.

Melanin. A skin pigment that gives skin its color. It acts as a sunscreen and protects the skin from absorbing too much vitamin D through ultraviolet light exposure. Sun-tanned skin and freckles are caused by melanin.

Melanoma. A skin cancer that develops in the skin cells that produce melanin. It can also occur inside the body, such as in the bowels or eyeball. It is a rare type of skin cancer but is the most deadly. It is due to uncontrolled growth of cells that create melanin.

Melatonin. A hormone produced by the brain's pineal gland during darkness but not during bright light. Melatonin is a derivative of serotonin and works with it to synchronize the body's sleep-wake cycle.

Osteomalacia. A condition where bones soften due to inadequate minerals. It is like rickets in children but occurs in adults. Symptoms include body pain, muscle weakness, and frail or brittle bones.

Osteoporosis. A condition of low bone mass and structural deterioration of bone tissue. Bones become fragile and fracture easily. Usually found in older women and men but can occur at all ages. Hip or vertebrae fracture is the most common result.

Parathyroid hormone. Made by the parathyroid glands, it controls the distribution of calcium and potassium in the body. It can move calcium out of the bone tissue and into the bloodstream.

Photoreceptor. A light-sensitive organ (like the eye), cell, or molecule that is stimulated by exposure to light.

Rickets. Disease in children where the bones do not form due to lack of vitamin D. Calcium is not deposited in the bone tissue because vitamin D is necessary to trigger the process. The bones are soft and bend easily, sometimes becoming misshapen, such as bowed legs.

Scurvy. Disease condition due to lack of vitamin C.

Squamous cell carcinoma. A common type of skin cancer occurring in late middle age and older. It is found mainly in areas exposed to sunlight, such as the nose and ears. It is more common in men than women and can be caused by sunlight or other environmental factors. Treatment is usually by surgical removal or targeted radiation.

Subclinical rickets. The disease has not progressed far enough for visible signs and symptoms in the patient. Children may have rickets, but it is not recognized early because their bones have not bent severely enough. By the time there is evidence of rickets, the condition has become severe.

Ultraviolet radiation. Ultraviolet light (UV) has invisible short-wavelength radiation that lies beyond the violet end of the visible spectrum. UV light has wavelengths between visible light and x-rays. Sunlight contains ultraviolet radiation.

UVA. Long-wavelength radiation that emits very little visible light. Ninety-eight percent of the sun's rays that reach earth are UVA type. UVA penetrates the skin but doesn't cause sunburn.

UVB. Medium wavelength radiation. This is the type of radiation the body needs in order to create vitamin D in the skin. Too much UVB can cause sunburn.

UVC. Short-wave high-energy rays. UVC is filtered out by the atmosphere. It can be used mechanically to disinfect pond water because of its germicidal property and will kill bacteria and algae.

ENDNOTES

INTRODUCTION

1. Gerard J. Tortora and Sandra Reynolds Grabowski, *Introduction to the Human Body* (New York: John Wiley & Sons, 2001), p. 490.

2. Ibid., p. 109.

3. Trevor G. Marshall, "Vitamin D Discovery Outpaces FDA Decision Making," *BioEssays* 30, no. 2 (January 15, 2008): 173–82.

4. Hector F. DeLuca, "Overview of General Physiologic Features and Functions of Vitamin D," *American Journal of Clinical Nutrition* 80, no. 6 (December 2004): 1689S–96S.

CHAPTER ONE

1. C. Scott Littleton, *Mythology: The Illustrated Anthology of World Myth & Storytelling* (London: Duncan Baird Publishers, 2002); Gwydion O'Hara, *Sun Lore: Folktales and Sagas from Around the World* (St. Paul: Llewellyn Publications, 1997), p. 26.

2. Joseph Campbell, *The Hero with a Thousand Faces* (Princeton, NJ: Princeton University Press, 1949), p. 58.

3. Jan F. Kreider, ed. in chief, and Frank Kreith, *Solar Energy Handbook* (New York: McGraw-Hill, 1981), pp. 1–4.

4. Soranus of Ephesus, *Diseases of Women*, trans. H. Lueneburg (Munich: J. H. Lehmann, 1894).

5. "Sun Worship," *Columbia Encyclopedia*, 6th ed. (New York: Columbia University Press, 2001).

6. Gordon J. Laing, *Survivals of Roman Religion* (New York: Longman, 1931), p. 192. Franz Cumont, *The Mysteries of Mithra*, trans. by Thomas J. McCormack (reprint; New York: Dover Publications, 1956), pp. 190–91. Frederick H. Cramer, *Astrology in Roman Law and Politics* (Philadelphia: American Philosophical Society, 1954), p. 4.

7. Madanjeet Singh, *The Sun: Symbol of Power and Life* (New York: Harry N. Abrams, 1993), pp. 26, 64.

8. Ibid., p. 180.

CHAPTER TWO

1. Victor E. Levine, "Sunlight and Its Many Values," *Scientific Monthly* 29, no. 6 (December 1929): 551–57.

2. Ibid., p. 552.

3. Jakob Lorber, *The Healing Power of Sunlight* (Salt Lake City: Merkur Publishing, 2000). First published 1851.

4. Ibid., p. 24.

5. In the late 1600s, Reverend Cotton Mather used the term "animalcules" to refer to the unknown but suspected microbes too small to see that were thought to be connected to disease. Cotton Mather, *The Angel of Bethesda*, ed. Gordon W. Jones (Barre, MA: American Antiquarian Society, 1972).

6. Philip E. Hockberger, "A History of Ultraviolet Photobiology for Humans, Animals and Microorganisms," *Photochemistry and Photobiology* 76, no. 6 (December 2002): 561–79.

7. Ibid.

8. Paul de Kruif, *Men against Death* (New York: Harcourt, Brace and Company, 1932), p. 287.

9. Richard Hobday, *The Healing Sun: Sunlight and Health in the Twenty-first Century* (London: Findhorn Press, 2000), p. 93.

10. De Kruif, *Men against Death*, p. 291.

11. Ibid., p. 297.

12. Ibid., p. 299.

13. Ibid., p. 319.

14. *Nobel Lectures, Physiology or Medicine 1901–1921* (Amsterdam: Elsevier Publishing Company, 1967). Online at http://nobelprize.org/medicine/laureates/1903/finsen-bio.html.

15. Ibid.; De Kruif, *Men against Death*, p. 299.

16. Charles Greeley Abbot, *The Sun and the Welfare of Man* (Washington, DC: Smithsonian Institution, 1929).

17. Levine, "Sunlight and its Many Values," pp. 551–57; De Kruif, *Men against Death*, p. 316.

18. De Kruif, *Men against Death*, p. 312.

19. Ibid., 349.

20. Janet Howell Clark, *Lighting in Relation to Public Health* (Baltimore: Williams and Wilkins Co., 1924), p. 137.

21. Levine, "Sunlight and its Many Values," p. 552.

22. Katharine Blunt and Ruth Cowan, *Ultraviolet Light and Vitamin D in Nutrition* (Chicago: University of Chicago Press, 1930), p. 30.

23. Philip E. Hockberger, "A History of Ultraviolet Photobiology for Humans, Animals and Microorganisms," *Photochemistry and Photobiology* 76, no. 6 (December 2002): 561–79.

24. Ibid., p. 565.

25. Jacob Liberman, *Light: Medicine of the Future* (Rochester, VT: Bear & Company, 1991), p. 141.

26. Levine, "Sunlight and its Many Values," p. 554.

27. Ibid., p. 556.

28. Ibid.

29. Ibid., p. 554.

30. Ibid., p. 557.

31. Blunt and Cowan, *Ultraviolet Light*, p. 211.

32. Hockberger, "A History of Ultraviolet Photobiology," p. 570.

CHAPTER THREE

1. Weston A. Price, *Nutrition and Physical Degeneration* (La Mesa, CA: Price-Pottenger Nutrition Foundation, 2003), p. 42.

2. Ibid., p. 41.

3. Ibid., p. 422.

4. Elmer Verner McCollum, *A History of Nutrition* (Boston: Houghton Mifflin, 1957), p. 266.

5. Casimir Funk, *Journal of State Medicine* 20 (1912): 341; McCollum, *A History of Nutrition*, p. 217.

6. Hector F. DeLuca, "Historical Overview," in *Vitamin D*, ed. F. H. Glorieux and D. Feldman (San Diego, CA: Academic Press, 1997), p. 3; Roy Porter, *The Greatest Benefit to Mankind* (New York: Norton, 1997), p. 551.

7. Elmer McCollum, *A History of Nutrition* (Boston: Houghton Mifflin, 1957), p. 195.

8. "History of Flaksted & Moskenes, Lofoten Islands, Norway," http://www.lofoten-info.no/history.htm#5 (accessed March 12, 2004).

9. E. V. McCollum and M. Davis. "The Necessity of Certain Lipins in the Diet during Growth," *Journal of Biological Chemistry* 15 (1915): 167–75.

10. Edward Mellanby, *A Story of Nutritional Research: The Effect of Some Dietary Factors on Bones and the Nervous System* (Baltimore: Williams and Wilkins Co., 1950), p. 3.

11. Jack W. Coburn and Nachman Brautbar, "Disease States in Man Related to Vitamin D," *Vitamin D: Molecular Biology and Clinical Nutrition*, ed. Anthony W. Norman (New York: Marcel Dekker, 1980), p. 529.

12. Edward Mellanby, "Progress in Medical Science," in James Jeans et al., *Scientific Progress*. Sir Halley Stewart lecture series (New York: Macmillan, 1936), p. 133.

13. Theobald A. Palm, "The Geographical Distribution and Etiology of Rickets," *Practitioner* (1890): 273.

14. Ibid., p. 279.

15. Ibid., pp. 279, 323.

16. Ibid., pp. 325, 328.

17. Ibid., p. 333.

18. Ibid., p. 342.

19. Edward Mellanby, *A Story of Nutritional Research: The Effect of Some Dietary Factors on Bones and the Nervous System* (Baltimore: Williams and Wilkins Company, 1950); Richard D. Semba. "Vitamin A as 'Anti-Infective' Therapy, 1920–1940," *Journal of Nutrition* 129 (1999): 783–91.

20. Mellanby, *A Story of Nutritional Research*, p. 13.

21. Mellanby, "Progress in Medical Science," p. 137.

22. E. C. McBeath and T. F. Zucker, "The Role of Vitamin D in the Control of Dental Caries in Children," *Journal of Nutrition* 15, no. 6 (1938): 547–64.

23. May Mellanby, "An Experimental Study of the Influence of Diet on Teeth Formation," *Lancet* (December 7, 1918): 767–70.

24. E. V. McCollum, N. Simmonds, J. E. Becker, and P.G. Shipley, "Studies on Experimental Rickets," *Journal of Biological Chemistry* 53 (1922): 293–312; Elmer Verner McCollum, *A History of Nutrition* (Boston: Houghton Mifflin, 1957), p. 276.

25. Mellanby, *A Story of Nutritional Research*, p. 209.

26. A. Sasson, Z. Etzion, S. Shany, G. M. Berlyne, and R. Yagil, "Growth and Bone Mineralisation as Affected by Dietary Calcium, Phytic Acid and Vitamin D," *Comparative Biochemistry and Physiology* 72, no. 1 (1982): 43–48.

27. C. H. Best and E. W. McHenry, "The Vitamins," *Canadian Medical Association Journal* (April 1930): 540–45.

28. Kurt Huldschinsky, "Preventive Irradiation of Children Against Rickets," *British Journal of Actinotherapy* (September 1928): 103–105.

29. Best and McHenry, "The Vitamins," pp. 540–45.

30. Katharine Blunt and Ruth Cowan, *Ultraviolet Light and Vitamin D in Nutrition* (Chicago: University of Chicago Press, 1930), p. 10.

31. Ibid., p. 126.

32. "Short-Wave Vitamins," *New York Times*, February 4, 1931, 24:4.

33. "Produced Vitamin D by an X-Ray Tube," *New York Times*, September 15, 1930, 3:4.

34. "Short-Wave Vitamins." *New York Times*.

35. "Vitamin D Rights Bought for Bread," *New York Times*, March 10, 1931, 21:6; "Produce New Bread with Vitamin D," *New York Times*, February 12, 1931, 2:5; "Mil-

lion Reported Bid for Vitamin D Rights," *New York Times*, February 13, 1931, 21:4; Rima D. Apple, "Patenting University Research," *ISIS* 80 (1989), 386.

36. Rima D. Apple, "Patenting University Research," *ISIS* 80 (1989): 387.

37. J. Waddell, "The Provitamin D of Cholesterol," *Journal of Biological Chemistry* 105 (July 1934): 711–39.

38. Blunt and Cowan, *Ultraviolet Light*, p. 131.

39. Ibid., p. 129.

40. Ibid., p. 139.

41. "Ultra-Violet Light Used to Enrich Food," *New York Times*, July 6, 1930, 14:8.

42. Blunt and Cowan, *Ultraviolet Light*, p. 146.

43. "Sees Child Health Rising," *New York Times*, March 19, 1932, 10:7.

CHAPTER FOUR

1. Reinhold Vieth, "The Pharmacology of Vitamin D, Including Fortification Strategies," in *Vitamin D*, 2nd ed., ed. David Feldman, Francis H. Glorieux, and J. Wesley Pike (San Diego: Academic Press, 1997), p. 1.

2. Reinhold Vieth, "Why 'Vitamin D' Is Not a Hormone, and Not a Synonym for 1,25-Dihydroxy-Vitamin D, Its Analogs or Deltanoids," *Journal of Steroid Biochemistry and Molecular Biology* 89–90 (2004): 571–73; A. J. Brown, C. S. Ritter, L. S. Holliday, J. C. Knutson, and S. A. Strugnell, "Tissue Distribution and Activity Studies of 1,24-Dihydroxyvitamin D2, a Metabolite of Vitamin D2 with Low Calcemic Activity in Vivo," *Biochemistry Pharmacology* 68, no. 7 (October 1, 2004): 1289–96; R. Lin and J. H. White, "The Pleiotropic Actions of Vitamin D," *Bioessays* 26, no. 1 (January 2004): 21–28; Hector F. DeLuca, "Overview of General Physiologic Features and Functions of Vitamin D," *American Journal of Clinical Nutrition* 80, no. 6 (December 2004): 1689S–96S.

3. R. S. Mason, "Vitamin D: New Insights into an Old Secosteroid," *Asia Pacific Journal of Clinical Nutrition* 14, suppl. (2005): S19; H. F. Deluca, "Vitamin D, the Vitamin and the Hormone," *Federation Proceedings* 33 (1974): 2211–19.

4. Reinhold Vieth, "Effects of Vitamin D on Bone and Natural Selection of Skin Color: How Much Vitamin D Nutrition are We Talking About?" *Bone Loss and Osteoporosis: An Anthropological Perspective*, ed. Sabrina C Agarwal and Sam D. Stout (New York: Kluwer Academic/Plenum Publishers, 2003), p. 145.

5. "Biochemistry and Physiology of Vitamin D," University of California-Riverside, Vitamin D Home Page, http://vitamind.ucr.edu/biochem.html (accessed December 14, 2005).

6. Reinhold Vieth, "Why 'Vitamin D' is Not a Hormone," pp. 571–573.

7. Rajiv Kumar, ed., *Vitamin D: Basic and Clinical Aspects* (Boson: Martinus Nijhoff Publishing, 1984), p. 29; Robert P. Heaney, "Functional Indices of Vitamin D Status and Ramifications of Vitamin D Deficiency," *American Journal of Clinical Nutrition* 80 suppl. (2004): 1706S–1709S.

8. J. J. Cannell, R. Vieth, J. C. Umhau, M. F. Holick, W. B. Grant, S. Madronich, C. F., Garland, and E. Giovannucci, "Epidemic Influenza and Vitamin D," *Epidemiology and Infection* 134, no. 6 (December 2006): 1129–40.

9. Elina Hypponen, Esa Laara, Antti Reunanen, Marjo-Riita Jarvelin, and Suvi M. Virtanen, "Intake of Vitamin D and Risk of Type 1 Diabetes: A Birth-Cohort Study," *Lancet* 358, no. 9292 (November 3, 2001): 1500–1503.

10. C. Mattila, P. Knekt, S. Mannisto, et al., "Serum 25-Hydroxyvitamin D Concentration and Subsequent Risk of Type 2 Diabetes," *Diabetes Care* 30 (2007): 2569–70.

11. Michael F. Holick, "Vitamin D Deficiency," *New England Journal of Medicine* 357, no. 3 (July 19, 2007): 266–81.

12. M. F. Holick, "Calcium and Vitamin D, Diagnostics and Therapeutics," *Clinical Laboratory Medicine* 20, no. 3 (September 2000): 569–90; "Vitamin D," Linus Pauling Institute's Micronutrient Information Center, Oregon State University, Corvallis, http://lpi.oregonstate.edu/infocenter/vitamins/vitaminD/ (accessed December 15, 2005).

13. John Cannell, "Vitamin D Newsletter," Vitamin D Council (July 2008).

14. "Vitamin D," Linus Pauling Institute's Micronutrient Information Center, Oregon State University.

15. R. Przybelski, S. Agrawal, D. Krueger, J. A. Engelke, F. Walbrun, and N. Binkley, "Rapid Correction of Low Vitamin D Status in Nursing Home Residents," *Osteoporosis International* (April 2008).

16. D. Chiricone, N. G. De Santo, and M. Cirillo, "Unusual Cases of Chronic Intoxication by Vitamin D," *Journal of Nephrology* 16, no. 6 (November/December 2003): 917–21.

17. V. Fulgoni, J. Nicholls, A. Reed, et. al., "Dairy Consumption and Related Nutrient Intake in African-American Adults and Children in the United States: Continuing Survey of Food Intakes by Individuals 1994–1996, 1998, and the National Health and Nutrition Examination Survey 1999–2000," *Journal of the American Dietetics Association* 107, no. 2 (February 2007): 256–64.

18. A. R. Webb and M. F. Holick, "The Role of Sunlight in the Cutaneous Production of Vitamin D_3," *Annual Reviews in Nutrition* 8 (1988): 375–99.

19. Mona S. Calvo, Susan J. Whiting, and Curtis N. Barton, "Vitamin D Fortification in the United States and Canada: Current Status and Data Needs," *American Journal of Clinical Nutrition* 80 suppl. (December 2004): 1710S–16S.

20. M. Brustad, T. Sandanger, L. Aksnes, and E. Lund, "Vitamin D Status in a Rural

Population of Northern Norway with High Fish Liver Consumption," *Public Health Nutrition* 7, no. 6 (September 2004): 783–99; S. J. Whiting and M. S. Calvo, "Dietary Recommendations for Vitamin D: A Critical Need for Functional End Points to Establish an Estimated Average Requirement," *Journal of Nutrition* 135, no. 2 (February 2005): 304–309.

21. S. E. Jolly, C. T. Eason, and C. Frampton, "Serum Calcium Levels in Response to Cholecalciferol and Calcium Carbonate in the Australian Brushtail Possum," *Pesticide Biochemistry Physiology* 47 (1993): 159–64; R. J. Henderson, C. M. Frampton, M. D. Thomas, and C. T. Eason, "Field Evaluations of Cholecalciferol, Gliftor, and Brodifacoum for the Control of Brushtail Possums (*Trichosurus vulpecula*)," New Zealand Plant Protection Society, http://www.hortnet.co/nx/publications/nzpps/proceedings/94/94_112.htm. International Relations and Security Network, Center for Security Studies, Zurich, Switzerland, http://www.isn.ethz.ch/researchpub/publihouse/za_cbw/docs/CBW127.htm.

22. Carla Morrow, "Cholecalciferol Poisoning," *Veterinary Medicine* (December 2001).

23. Chiricone, De Santa, and Cirillo, "Unusual Cases of Chronic Intoxication by Vitamin D," pp. 917–21.

24. Ronald L. Horst and Timothy A. Reinhardt, "Vitamin D Metabolism," in *Vitamin D*, 2nd ed., ed. David Feldman, Francis H. Glorieux, and J. Wesley Pike (San Diego: Academic Press, 1997), pp. 13–31.

25. T. M. Sandanger, M. Brustad, E. Lund, and I. C. Burkow, "Change in Levels of Persistent Organic Pollutants in Human Plasma after Consumption of a Traditional Northern Norwegian Fish Dish—Molje (Cod, Cod Liver, Cod Liver Oil and Hard Roe)," *Journal of Environmental Monitoring* 5, no. 1 (February 2003): 160–65.

26. Mark Kurlansky, *Cod: A Biography of the Fish That Changed the World* (New York: Penguin, 1997); "Carping Kills Cod," *New Scientist* (January 2006): 4.

27. W. S. Van de Ven, "Mercury and Selenium in Cod-Liver Oil," *Clinical Toxicology* 12, no. 5 (1978): 579–81.

28. Terhi A. Lutila et al., "Bioavailability of Vitamin D from Wild Edible Mushrooms (*Cantharellus tubaeformis*) as Measured with a Human Bioassay," *American Journal of Clinical Nutrition* 69 (1999): 95–98.

29. Paul Stamets, personal interview on February 22, 2005; Paul Stamets, *Mycelium Running* (Berkeley, CA: Ten Speed Press, 2005).

30. Paul Stamets, personal interview.

31. John S. Roberts et al., "Vitamin D_2 Formation from Post-Harvest UV-B Treatment of Mushrooms (*Agaricus bisporus*) and Retention During Storage," *Journal of Agricultural Food Chemistry* 56, no. 12 (2008): 4541–44; Anja Teichmann et al., "Sterol and Vitamin D_2 Concentrations in Cultivated and Wild Grown Mushrooms: Effects of UV Irradiation," *Food Science and Technology* 40, no. 5 (June 2007): 815–22.

32. Anna-Mari Natri et al., "Bread Fortified with Cholecalciferol Increases the Serum 25-Hydroxyvitamin D Concentration in Women as Effectively as a Cholecalciferol Supplement," *Journal of Nutrition* 136 (2006): 123–27.

33. Mary G. Enig, *Know Your Fats: The Complete Primer for Understanding the Nutrition of Fats, Oils, and Cholesterol* (Silver Spring, MD: Bethesda Press, 2004), p. 71.

34. Connie Leas, *Fat: It's Not What You Think* (Amherst, NY: Prometheus Books, 2008).

35. J. S. Vobecky, J. Vobecky, and L. Normand, "Risk and Benefit of Low Fat Intake in Childhood," *Annals of Nutrition and Metabolism* 39, no. 2 (1995): 124–33; S. R. Dunn-Emke, G. Weidner, E. B. Peggengill, R. O. Marlin, C. Chi, and D. M. Ornish, "Nutrient Adequacy of a Very Low-Fat Vegan Diet," *Journal of the American Dietetics Association* 105, no. 9 (September 2005): 1442–46; L. J. Deftos, M. M. Miller, and D. W. Burton, "A High-Fat Diet Increases Calcitonin Secretion in the Rat," *Bone and Mineral* 5, no. 3 (March 1989): 303–308.

36. Leas, *Fat: It's Not What You Think*.

37. Frank B. Hu, Meir J. Stampfer, JoAnn E. Manson, et al., "Dietary Fat Intake and the Risk of Coronary Heart Disease in Women," *New England Journal of Medicine* 337, no. 21 (November 20, 1997): 1491–99.

38. Claudia M. Grieser, Eberhard M. Greiser, and Martina Doren, "Menopausal Hormone Therapy and Risk of Ovarian Cancer: A Systematic Review," *Human Reproduction Update* 13, no. 5 (September/October 3007): 453–63.

39. "Dietary Supplement Fact Sheet: Vitamin D, Office of Dietary Supplements, National Institutes of Health," http://ods.nih.gov/factsheets/vitamind.asp (accessed October 10, 2008).

40. Lesley E. Rhodes, Brian H. Durham, William D. Fraser, and Peter S. Friedmann, "Dietary Fish Oil Reduces Basal and Ultraviolet B-Generated PGE_2 Levels in Skin and Increases the Threshold to Provocation of Polymorphic Light Eruption," *Journal of Investigative Dermatology* 105, no. 4 (October 1995): 532–35.

41. Mona S. Calvo and Susan J. Whiting, "Overview of the Proceedings from Experimental Biology 2004 Symposium: Vitamin D Insufficiency: A Significant Risk Factor in Chronic Disease and Potential Disease-Specific Biomarkers of Vitamin D Sufficiency," *Journal of Nutrition* 135, no. 2 (February 2005): 301–303; Mona S. Calvo, Susan J. Whiting, and Curtis N. Barton, "Vitamin D Intake: A Global Perspective of Current Status," *Journal of Nutrition* 135, no. 2 (February 2005): 310–17; Charles Marwick, "New Light on Skin Cancer Mechanisms," *Journal of the American Medical Association* 274, no. 6 (August 9, 1995): 445–46.

42. S. J. Whiting and M. S. Calvo, "Dietary Recommendations for Vitamin D: A Critical Need for Functional End Points to Establish an Estimated Average Requirement," *Journal of Nutrition* 135, no. 2 (February 2005): 304–309. Rhodes, Durham,

Fraser, and Friedmann, "Dietary Fish Oil Reduces Basal and Ultraviolet B-Generated PGE$_2$ Levels in Skin."

43. K. Rajakumar and S. B. Thomas, "Reemerging Nutritional Rickets: A Historical Perspective," *Archives of Pediatric Adolescent Medicine* 159, no. 4 (April 2005): 335–41; T. Henriksen, A. Dahlback, S. H. Larsen, and J. Moan, "Ultraviolet-radiation and Skin Cancer. Effect of an Ozone Layer Depletion," *Photochemistry and Photobiology* 51, no. 5 (May 1990): 579–82.

44. C. G. Miller and W. Chutkan, "Vitamin-D Deficiency Rickets in Jamaican Children," *Archives of Disease in Childhood* 51, no. 3 (March 1976): 214–18; Kathleen E. Fuller, "Health Disparities: Reframing the Problem," *Medical Science Monitor* 9, no. 3 special report (March 2003): SR9–15.

45. Fuller, "Health Disparities: Reframing the Problem."

46. Mona S. Calvo, Susan J. Whiting, and Curtis N. Barton, "Vitamin D Intake: A Global Perspective of Current Status," *Journal of Nutrition* 135, no. 2 (February 2005): 310–17.

47. Marianne Berwick, Bruce K. Armstrong, Leah Ben-Porat, et al., "Sun Exposure and Mortality from Melanoma," *Journal of the National Cancer Institute* 97, no. 3 (February 2, 2005): 195–99; R. S. Mason, "Vitamin D: New Insights into an Old Secosteroid," *Asia Pacific Journal of Clinical Nutrition* 14, suppl. (2005): S19; K. M. Dixon, S. S. Deo, G. Wong, et al., "Skin Cancer Prevention: A Possible Role of 1,25dihydroxyvitamin D and Its Analogs," *Journal of Steroid Biochemistry and Molecular Biology* 97, nos. 1–2 (October 2005): 137–43; A. M. Hughes, B. K. Armstrong, C. M. Vajdic, et al., "Sun Exposure May Protect against Non-Hodgkin Lymphoma: A Case-Control Study," *International Journal of Cancer* 112, no. 5 (December 10, 2004): 865–71, Kathryn Z. Guyton, Thomas W. Kensler, and Gary H. Posner, "Vitamin D and Vitamin D Analogs as Cancer Chemopreventive Agents," *Nutrition Reviews* 61, no. 7 (July 2003): 227–37. G. G. Schwartz, "Vitamin D and the Epidemiology of Prostate Cancer," *Seminars in Dialysis* 18, no. 4 (July/August 2005): 276–89.

48. Berwick, Armstrong, Ben-Porat et al., "Sun Exposure and Mortality from Melanoma."

49. Paul Affleck, "Sun Exposure and Health," *Nursing Standard* 19, no. 47 (August 3–9, 2005): 50–55.

50. Mortality rate maps for skin, breast, and prostate cancer, courtesy of the National Cancer Institute, are available at http://www.3.cancer.gov/atlasplus (accessed December 12, 2008); A. Zittermann, "Vitamin D in Preventive Medicine: Are We Ignoring the Evidence?" *British Journal of Nutrition* 89, no. 5 (May 2003): 552–72; Alex Vasquez, Gilbert Manso, and John Cannell, "The Clinical Importance of Vitamin D (Cholecalciferol): A Paradigm Shift with Implications for all Healthcare Providers," *Alternative Therapies* 10, no. 5 (September/October 2004): 28–36.

51. "'Guardian of the Genome' Protein Found to Underlie Skin Tanning," Dana-Farber Cancer Institute, Harvard Medical School, press release, March 8, 2007.

52. M. L. Melamed, E. D. Michos, W. Post, and B. Astor, "25-Hydroxyvitamin D Levels and the Risk of Mortality in the General Population," *Archives of Internal Medicine* 168, no. 15 (August 11, 2008): 1629–37.

53. A. Zittermann, "Vitamin D in Preventive Medicine: Are We Ignoring the Evidence?" *British Journal of Nutrition* 89, no. 5 (May 2003): 552–72; Vasquez, Manso, and Cannell, "The Clinical Importance of Vitamin D (Cholecalciferol)."

CHAPTER FIVE

1. Centers for Disease Control, "Severe Malnutrition among Young Children; Georgia, January 1977–June 1999," *MMWR Weekly* 50, no. 12 (March 30, 2001): 224–27.

2. "D-Ficiency," *Vegetarian Times* 322 (June 2004): 13; D. Rucker, J. A. Allan, G. H. Fick, and D. A. Hanley, "Vitamin D Insufficiency in a Population of Healthy Western Canadians," *Canadian Medical Association Journal* 166, no. 12 (2002): 1517–24; Daniel J. Raiten and Mary Frances Picciano, "Vitamin D and Health in the 21st Century: Bone and Beyond," executive summary, *American Journal of Clinical Nutrition* 80 suppl. (2004): 1673S–77S.

3. Mona S. Calvo and Susan J. Whiting, "Overview of the Proceedings from Experimental Biology 2004 Symposium: Vitamin D Insufficiency: A Significant Risk Factor in Chronic Diseases and Potential Disease-Specific Biomarkers of Vitamin D Sufficiency," *Journal of Nutrition* 135, no. 2 (February 2005): 301–303; E. M. Haney, D. Stadler, and M. M. Bliziotes, "Vitamin D Insufficiency in Internal Medicine Residents," *Calcified Tissue International* 76, no. 1 (January 2005): 11–16.

4. William A. Stini, "Bone Loss, Fracture Histories, and Body Composition," in *Bone Loss and Osteoporosis: An Anthropological Perspective*, ed. Sabrina C. Agarwal and Sam D. Stout (New York: Kluwer Academic/Plenum Press, 2003), pp. 63–89.

5. N. J. Shaw and B. R. Pal, "Vitamin D Deficiency in UK Asian Families: Activating a New Concern," *Archives of Disease in Childhood* 86 (2002): 147–49; Alok Sachan, Renu Gupta, Vinita Das, Anjoo Agarwal, Pradeep K. Awasthi, and Vijayalakshmi Bahtia, "High Prevalence of Vitamin D Deficiency among Pregnant Women and Their Newborns in Northern India," *American Journal of Clinical Nutrition* 81, no. 5 (May 2005): 1060–64; S. H. Sedrani, A. W. Alidrissy, and K. M. El Arabi, "Sunlight and Vitamin D Status in Normal Saudi Subjects," *American Journal of Clinical Nutrition* 38, no. 1 (July 1983): 129–32; S. H. Sedrani, "Low 25-Hydroxyvitamin D and Normal

Serum Calcium Cconcentrations in Saudi Arabia: Riyadh Region," *Annals of Nutrition and Metabolism* 28, no. 3 (1984): 181–85; S. H. Sedrani, "Vitamin D Status of Saudi Men," *Tropical and Geographical Medicine* 36, no. 2 (June 1984): 181–87.

6. T. D. Thacher, P. R. Fischer, J. M. Pettifor, J. O. Lawson, C. O. Isichei, J. C. Reding, and G. M. Chan, "A Comparison of Calcium, Vitamin D, or Both for Nutritional Rickets in Nigerian Children," *New England Journal of Medicine* 341, no. 8 (August 1999): 563–68; J. M. Pettifor, P. Ross, and J. Wang, "Rickets in Children of Rural Origin in South Africa: Is Dietary Calcium a Factor?" *Journal of Pediatrics* 92, no. 2 (1978): 320–24; G. Kutluk, F. Cetinkaya, and M. Basak, "Comparisons of Oral Calcium, High Dose Vitamin D and a Combination of These in the Treatment of Nutritional Rickets in Children," *Journal of Tropical Pediatrics* 48, no. 6 (2002): 351–53.

7. Elizabeth A. C. Sellers, Atul Sharma, and Celia Rodd, "Adaptation of Inuit Children to a Low-Calcium Diet," *Canadian Medical Association Journal* 168, no. 9 (April 29, 2003): 1141–43.

8. Sachan et al., "High Prevalence of Vitamin D Deficiency among Pregnant Women and Their Newborns in Northern India"; Sedrani, Alidrissy, and El Arabi, "Sunlight and Vitamin D Status in Normal Saudi Subjects"; Sedrani, "Low 25-Hydroxyvitamin D and Normal Serum Calcium Concentrations in Saudi Arabia: Riyadh Region"; Sedrani, "Vitamin D Status of Saudi Men."

9. Thacher et al., "A Comparison of Calcium, Vitamin D, or Both for Nutritional Rickets in Nigerian Children"; Pettifor, Ross, and Wang, "Rickets in Children of Rural Origin in South Africa"; Kutluk, Cetinkaya, and Basak, "Comparisons of Oral Calcium, High Dose Vitamin D and a Combination of These in the Treatment of Nutritional Rickets in Children."

10. Sellers, Sharma, and Rodd, "Adaptation of Inuit Children to a Low-Calcium Diet."

11. Price, *Nutrition and Physical Degeneration*.

12. D. M. Large, E. B. Mawer, and M. Davies, "Dystrophic Calcification, Cataracts, and Enamel Hypoplasia Due to Long-Standing, Privational Vitamin D Deficiency," *Metabolic Bone Disease Related Research* 5, no. 5 (1984): 215–18.

13. L. W. Mayron, J. N. Ott, E. J. Amontree, and R. Nations, "Light, Radiation, and Dental Caries," *Academic Therapy* 10 (1975): 441–48. The same authors published "Caries Reduction in School Children," *Applied Radiology* (July/August 1975): 56–58.

14. E. C. McBeath and T. F. Zucker, "The Role of Vitamin D in the Control of Dental Caries in Children," *Journal of Nutrition* 15, no. 6 (1938): 547–64; B. East, "Mean Annual Hours of Sunshine and the Incidence of Dental Caries," *American Journal of Public Health* 29 (1939): 777–80; N. B. Palmer and J. D. Palmer, "The Dental Caries Experience of 5-, 12- and 14-Year-Old Children in Great Britain," surveys coordinated by the British Association for the Study of Community Dentistry in 1990–91, 1991–92, and 1992–93, *Community Dental Health* 11, no. 1 (1994): 42–52.

15. Lindsey Tanner, "More Americans are Getting Osteoporosis," *Seattle Times*, July 26, 2004; Reinhold Vieth, "The Pharmacology of Vitamin D, Including Fortification Strategies," *Vitamin D* (1997): 4; B. Dawson-Hughes, G. E. Dallal, E. A. Krall, S. Harris, L. J. Sokoll, and G. Falconer, "Effect of Vitamin D Supplementation on Wintertime and Overall Bone Loss in Healthy Postmenopausal Women," *Annals of Internal Medicine* 115 (1991): 505–12.

16. P. Kannus, K. Uusi-Rasi, M. Palvanen, and J. Parkkari, "Non-Pharmacological Means to Prevent Fractures among Older Adults," *Annals of Medicine* 37, no. 4 (2005): 303–10; L. Flicker, R. Macinnis, M. Stein, S. Scherer, K. Mead, and C. Nowson, "Vitamin D to Prevent Falls in Older People in Residential Care," *Asia Pacific Journal of Clinical Nutrition* 14, suppl. (2005): S18; H. A. Bischoff-Ferrari, W. C. Willett, J. B. Wong, E. Giovannucci, T. Dietrich, and B. Dawson-Hughes, "Fracture Prevention with Vitamin D Supplementation: A Meta-analysis of Randomized Controlled Trials," *Journal of the American Medical Association* 293, no. 18 (May 2005): 2257–64.

17. I. Kawasaki, "Intake of Vitamin D and Muscular Volume," *Clinical Calcium* 15, no. 9 (September 2005): 1517–21; I. Endo and D. Inoue, "Effect of Calcium and Vitamin D on Skeletal Muscle," *Clinical Calcium* 13, no. 7 (July 2003): 905–907; L. Dukas, H. B. Staehelen, E. Schacht, and H. A. Bischoff, "Better Functional Mobility in Community-Dwelling Elderly is Related to D-Hormone Serum Levels and to Daily Calcium Intake," *Journal of Nutrition Health and Aging* 9, no. 5 (September/October 2005): 347–51.

18. A. Goulding et al., "Children Who Avoid Drinking Cow's Milk Are at Increased Risk for Prepubertal Bone Fractures," *Journal of the American Dietetic Association* 104, no. 2 (2004): 250–53; "'Calcium Crisis' Affects American Youth," www.nichd .nih.gov/new/releases/calcium_crisis.cfm?from=milk (accessed December 10, 2001).

19. Endo and Inoue, "Effect of Calcium and Vitamin D on Skeletal Muscle."

20. P. Ko, R. Burkert, J. McGrath, and D. Eyles, "Maternal Vitamin D(3) Deprivation and the Regulation of Apoptosis and Cell Cycle during Rat Brain Development," *Developmental Brain Research* 153, no. 1 (October 15, 2004): 61–86.

21. J. McGrath, "Does 'Imprinting' with Low Prenatal Vitamin D Contribute to the Risk of Various Adult Disorders?" *Medical Hypotheses* 56, no. 3 (March 2001): 367–71; A. Mackay-Sim, F. Feron, D. Eyles, T. Burne, and J. McGrath, "Schizophrenia, Vitamin D, and Brain Development," *International Review of Neurobiology* 59 (2004): 351–80; I. S. Wincherts, N. M. van Schoor, et al., *Journal of Clinical Endocrine Metabolism* 92, no. 6 (June 2007): 2058–65; Darryl W. Eyles, J. Brown, et al., "Vitamin D3 and Brain Development," *Neuroscience* 118, no. 3 (2003): 641–53; Axel Becker, Darryl W. Eyles, John J. McGrath, and Gisela Grecksch, "Transient Prenatal Vitamin D Deficiency is Associated with Subtle Alternations in Learning and Memory Functions in Adult Rats," *Behavioural Brain Research* 161, no. 2 (June 20, 2005): 306–12.

22. John Cannell, "Autism and Vitamin D," *Medical Hypotheses* (October 4, 2007).

23. John McGrath, K. Saari, H. Hakko, J. Jokelainen, P. Jones, M. R. Jarvelin, D. Chant, and M. Isohanni, "Vitamin D Supplementation during the First Year of Life and Risk of Schizophrenia: A Finnish Birth Cohort Study," *Schizophrenia Research* 67, nos. 2–3 (April 1, 2004): 237–45.

24. A. Mackay-Sim, F. Feron, D. Eyles, T. Burne, and J. McGrath, "Schizophrenia, Vitamin D, and Brain Development," *International Reviews in Neurobiology* 59 (2004): 351–80.

25. R. P. Martin, P. Foels, G. Clanton, and K. Moon, "Season of Birth is Related to Child Retention Rates, Achievement, and Rate of Diagnosis of Specific LD," *Journal of Learning Disabilities* 37, no. 4 (July/August 2004): 307–17; J. J. McGrath, S. Saha, D. E. Lieberman, and S. Buka, "Season of Birth Is Associated with Anthropometric and Neurocognitive Outcomes during Infancy and Childhood in a General Population Birth Cohort," *Schizophrenia Research* 81, no. 1 (January 2006): 91–100; Margaret M. Halleran, "The Effect of Rickets on the Mental Development of Young Children," *Archives of Psychology* (July 1938); John McGrath, Darryl Eyles, B. Mowry, R. Yolken, and S. Buka, "Low Maternal Vitamin D as a Risk Factor for Schizophrenia; A Pilot Study Using Banked Sera," *Schizophrenia Research* 63, nos. 1–2 (September 1, 2003): 73–78.

26. Sukru Hatun, Behzat Ozkan, Zerrin Orbak, et al., "Vitamin D Deficiency in Early Infancy," *Journal of Nutrition* 135 (February 2005): 279–82; A. Dawodu and C. L. Wagner, "Mother-Child Vitamin D Deficiency: An International Perspective," *Archives of Disease in Childhood* 92, no. 9 (September 1, 2007): 737–40.

27. D. Eyles, J. Brown, A. Mackay-Sim, et al., "Vitamin D3 and Brain Development," *Neuroscience* 118, no. 3 (2003): 641–53.

28. Halleran, "The Effect of Rickets on the Mental Development of Young Children."

29. A. S. Brown and E. S. Susser, "Prenatal Nutritional Deficiency and Risk of Adult Schizophrenia," *Schizophrenia Bulletin* 34, no. 6 (August 4, 2008).

30. M. T. Pugliese, D. L. Blumberg, J. Hudzinski, and S. Kay, "Nutritional Rickets in Suburbia," *Journal of American College of Nutrition* 17, no. 6 (December 1998): 637–41; Valerie Fildes, *Wet Nursing: A History from Antiquity to the Present* (New York: Basil Blackwell, 1988), pp. 222–28.

31. W. E. Stumph, "Vitamin D and the Digestive System," *European Journal of Drug Metabolism and Pharmacokinetics* 33, no. 2 (April/June 2008): 85–100.

32. C. M. Schulte, "Review Article: Bone Disease in Inflammatory Bowel Disease," *Alimentary Pharmacology Therapy* 20, suppl. 4 (October 2004): 43–49; L. M. Cruse, J. Valeriano, F. B. Vasey, and J. D. Carter, "Prevalence of Evaluation and Treatment of Glucocorticoid-Induced Osteoporosis in Men," *Journal of Clinical Rheumatology* 12, no. 5 (October 2006): 221–25; American College of Rheumatology Ad Hoc Committee

on Glucocorticoid-Induced Osteoporosis, "Recommendations for the Prevention and Treatment of Glucocorticoid-Induced Osteoporosis: 2001 Update," *Arthritis and Rheumatism* 44, no. 7 (July 2001): 1496–1503.

33. Norma Peterson, "The Sunshine Factor: Vitamin D and Breast Cancer," *Breast Cancer Action Network Newsletter* (June 1992): 12; William B. Grant, "An Ecologic Study of Dietary and Solar Ultraviolet-B Links to Breast Carcinoma Mortality Rates," *Cancer* 94, no. 1 (January 1, 2002): 272–81; A. J. Brown, C. S. Ritter, L. S. Holliday, et al., "Tissue Distribution and Activity Studies of 1,24-dihydroxyvitamin D2, a Metabolite of Vitamin D2 with Low Calcemic Activity in Vivo," *Biochemical Pharmacology* 68, no. 7 (October 1, 2004): 1289–96; P. A. Hershberger, R. A. Modzelewski, Z. R. Shurin, et al., "1,25-Dihydroxycholecalciferol (1,25-D3) Inhibits the Growth of Squamous Cell Carcinoma and Down-Modulates p21Waf1/Cip1 in Vitro and in Vivo," *Cancer Research* 59, no. 11 (June 1, 1999): 2644–49; E. D. Gorham, F. C. Garland, and C. F. Garland, "Sunlight and Breast Cancer Incidence in the U.S.S.R.," *International Journal of Epidemiology* 19 (1990): 820–24.

34. R. Lin, and J. H. White, "The Pleiotropic Actions of Vitamin D," *Bioessays* 26, no. 1 (January 26, 2004): 21–28; Cedric F. Garland, Frank C. Garland, and Edward D. Gorham, "Calcium and Vitamin D: Their Potential Roles in Colon and Breast Cancer Prevention," *Annals of the New York Academy of Sciences* 889 (1999): 107–19; G. P. Studzinski and D. C. Moore, "Sunlight—Can It Prevent as Well as Cause Cancer?" *Cancer Research* 55, no. 18 (1995): 4014–22; D. Bodiwala, C. J. Luscombe, M. E. French, et al., "Susceptibility to Prostate Cancer: Studies on Interactions between UVR Exposure and Skin Type," *Carcinogenesis* 24, no. 4 (April 1, 2003): 711–17; Coleman Gross, Donna M. Peehl, and David Feldman, "Vitamin D and Prostate Cancer," in *Vitamin D*, ed. D. Feldman, F. H. Glorieux, and J. W. Pike (San Deigo: Academic Press, 1999), p. 1126.

35. Mortality rate maps for skin, breast, and prostate cancer, courtesy of the National Cancer Institute, are available at http://www.3.cancer.gov/atlasplus (accessed December 12, 2008); Garland, Garland, and Gorham, "Calcium and Vitamin D"; Peterson, "The Sunshine Factor"; S. J. Moon, A. A. Fryer, and R. C. Strange, "Ultraviolet Radiation, Vitamin D and Prostate Cancer Risk," *Photochemistry and Photobiology* (January 1, 2005); D. M. Freedman, M. Dosemeci, and K. McGlynn, "Sunlight and Mortality from Breast, Ovarian, Colon, Prostate, and Non-Melanoma Skin Cancer: A Composite Death Certificate Based Case-Control Study," *Occupational and Environmental Medicine* 59 (2002): 257–62.

36. T. C. Chen and M. F. Holick, "Vitamin D and Prostate Cancer Prevention and Treatment," *Trends in Endocrinology and Metabolism* 14, no. 9 (November 2003): 423–30.

37. Cedric F. Garland, "More on Preventing Skin Cancer," *British Medical Journal* 327 (December 22, 2003): 1228; Garland, Garland, and Gorham, "Calcium and Vitamin D."

38. B. Peplonska, J. Lissowska, T. J. Hartman, et. al., "Adulthood Lifetime Physical Activity and Breast Cancer," *Epidemiology* 19, no. 2 (March 2008): 226–36.

39. Marilynn Larkin, "How Green Is Your Workout?" *Lancet* 355 (2000): 1702–1703.

40. Diane M. Harris and Vay Liang W. Go, "Vitamin D and Colon Carcinogenesis," *Journal of Nutrition* 134, suppl. (December 2004): 3463S–71S; Diane Feskanich, Jing Ma, and Charles S. Fuchs, "Plasma Vitamin D Metabolites and Risk of Colorectal Cancer in Women," *Cancer Epidemiology Biomarkers & Prevention* 13 (September 2004): 1502–1508; E. Cho, S. A. Smith-Warner, D. Spiegelman, et al., "Dairy Foods, Calcium, and Colorectal Cancer: A Pooled Analysis of 10 Cohort Studies," *Journal of the National Cancer Institute* 96, no. 13 (July 1996): 1015–22.

41. C. F. Garland and F. C. Garland, "Do Sunlight and Vitamin D Reduce the Likelihood of Colon Cancer?" *International Journal of Epidemiology* 9 (1980): 227–31; Diane Feskanich, Jing Ma, Charles S. Fuchs, et al., "Plasma Vitamin D Metabolites and Risk of Colorectal Cancer in Women," *Cancer Epidemiology Biomarkers and Prevention* 13 (September 2004): 1502–1508; Harris and Go, "Vitamin D and Colon Carcinogenesis."

42. E. S. Lefkowitz and C. F. Garland, "Sunlight, Vitamin D, and Ovarian Cancer Mortality Rates in U.S. Women," *International Journal of Epidemiology* 23 (1994): 1133–36.

43. T. R. Fears, C. C. Bird, D. Guerry, R. W. Sagebiel, M. H. Gail, D. E. Elder, A. Halpern, E. A. Holly, P. Hartge, and M. A. Tucker, "Average UVB Flux and Time Outdoors Predict Melanoma Risk," *Cancer Research* 62, no. 14 (July 15, 2002): 3992–96; "Global Cancer Statistics, 2002," *CA: Cancer Journal for Clinicians* 55, no. 2 (2005): 74–108.

44. E. Hypponen, E. Laara, A. Reunanen, M. R. Jarvelin, and S. M. Virtanen, "Intake of Vitamin D and Risk of Type 1 Diabetes: A Birth-Cohort Study," *Lancet* 358, no. 9292 (November 3, 2001): 1500–1503; Oliver Gillie, *Sunlight Robbery* (London: Health Research Forum, 2004), p. 16.

45. E. Hypponen, "Micronutrients and the Risk of Type 1 Diabetes: Vitamin D, Vitamin E, and Nicotinamide," *Nutrition Review* 62, no. 9 (September 2004): 340–47; Hypponen et al., "Intake of Vitamin D and Risk of Type 1 Diabetes."

46. G. Ulett, "Geographic Distribution of Multiple Sclerosis," *Diseases of the Nervous System* 9 (1948): 342–46.

47. Anne-Louise Ponsonby, Anthony McMichael, and Ingrid van der Mei, "Ultraviolet Radiation and Autoimmune Disease: Insights from Epidemiological Research," *Toxicology* 181–82 (2002): 71–78; K. L. Munger, S. M. Zhang, E. O'Reilly, et al., "Vitamin D Intake and Incidence of Multiple Sclerosis," *Neurology* 62 (January 2004): 60–65.

48. C. E. Hayes, "Vitamin D: A Natural Inhibitor of Multiple Sclerosis," *Proceedings of Nutrition Society* 59, no. 4 (2000): 531–35.

49. Ponsonby, McMichael, and van der Mei, "Ultraviolet Radiation and Autoimmune Disease."

50. Ibid.

51. Gregory A. Plotnikoff and Joanna M. Quigley, "Prevalence of Severe Hypovitaminosis D in Patients with Persistent, Nonspecific Musculoskeletal Pain," *Mayo Clinic Proceedings* 78, no. 12 (December 2003); R. Mascarenhas and S. Mobarhan, "Hypovitaminosis D-Induced Pain," *Nutrition Reviews* 62, no. 9 (September 2004): 354–59.

52. Joan Schwartz, "Research Briefs," *Boston University Bridge* (May 15, 2003); Mascarenhas and Mobarhan, "Hypovitaminosis D-Induced Pain."

53. S. L. Bowyer and J. R. Hollister, "Limb Pain in Childhood," *Pediatric Clinics of North America* 31, no. 5 (October 1984): 1053–81; L. Kohnen and J. Magotteaux, "Acute and Recurrent Night Leg Pain in Young Children: 'Growing Pains,'" *Revue Medical de Liege* 59, no. 6 (June 2004): 363–66; A. M. Evans and S. D. Scutter, "Prevalence of 'Growing Pains' in Young Children," *Journal of Pediatrics* 145, no. 2 (August 2004): 255–58; P. Manners, "Are Growing Pains a Myth?" *Australian Family Physician* 28, no. 2 (February 1999): 124–27.

54. Manners, "Are Growing Pains a Myth?"; F. Oberklaid, D. Amos, C. Liu, F. Jarman, A. Sanson, and M. Prior, "Growing Pains: Clinical and Behavioral Correlates in a Community Sample," *Journal of Developmental and Behavioral Pediatrics* 18, no. 2 (April 1997): 102–106.

55. Evans and Scutter, "Prevalence of 'Growing Pains' in Young Children"; Gillie, *Sunlight Robbery*, p. 18.

56. H. A. Peterson, "Leg Aches," *Pediatric Clinics of North America* 24, no. 4 (November 1977): 731–36.

57. J. J. Calabro, A. E. Wachtel, W. B. Holgerson, and M. M. Repice, "Growing Pains: Fact or Fiction?" *Postgraduate Medicine* 59, no. 2 (February 1976): 66–72; S. R. Weiner, "Growing Pains," *American Family Physician* 27, no. 1 (January 1983): 189–91.

58. Angelo P. Giardino, "Fibromyalgia," E Medicine/WebMD, http://www.emedicine.com/ped/topic777.htm (accessed May 16, 2006).

59. T. J. Romano, "Fibromyalgia in Children; Diagnosis and Treatment," *West Virginia Medical Review* 87, no. 3 (March 1991): 112–14.

60. S. Arunabh, S. Pollack, J. Yeh, and J. F. Aloia, "Body Fat Content and 25-Hydroxyvitamin D Levels in Healthy Women," *Journal of Clinical Endocrinology and Metabolism* 88, no. 1 (January 2003): 157–61; Elena Kamycheva, Ragnar M. Joakimsen and Rolf Jorde, "Intakes of Calcium and Vitamin D Predict Body Mass Index in the Population of Northern Norway," *Journal of Nutrition* 133 (January 2003): 102–106.

61. Sarina Schrager, "Dietary Calcium Intake and Obesity," *Journal of American Board of Family Practice* 18 (2005): 205–10. Kamycheva, Joakimsen, and Jorde,

"Intakes of Calcium and Vitamin D Predict Body Mass Index in the Population of Northern Norway"; W. C. Ping-Delfos et al., "Acute Suppression of Spontaneous Food Intake Following Dairy Calcium and Vitamin D," *Asian Pacific Journal of Clinical Nutrition* 13, suppl. (2004): S82, funded by Dairy Australia. Michael B. Zemel, et al., "Regulation of Adiposity by Dietary Calcium," *FASEB Journal* 14 (2000): 1132–38, funded by the National Dairy Council.

62. M. F. McCarty and C. A. Thomas, "PTH Excess May Promote Weight Gain by Impeding Catecholamine-Induced Lipolysis—Implications for the Impact of Calcium, Vitamin D, and Alcohol on Body Weight," *Medical Hypotheses* 61, nos. 5–6 (November/December 2003): 535–42; E. Kamycheva, J. Sundsfjord, and R. Jorde, "Serum Parathyroid Hormone Level Is Associated with Body Mass Index. The 5th Tromso Study," *European Journal of Endochronology* 151, no. 2 (August 2004): 167–72; N. Hamoui, G. Anthone, and P. F. Crooks, "Calcium Metabolism in the Morbidly Obese," *Obesity Surgery* 14, no. 1 (January 2004): 9–12.

63. P. E. Norman and J. T. Powell, "Vitamin D, Shedding Light on the Development of Disease in Peripheral Arteries," *Arteriosclerosis, Thrombosis, and Vascular Biology* 25 (2005): 39.

64. L. B. Tanko, Y. Z. Bagger, and C. Christiansen, "Low Bone Mineral Density in the Hip as a Marker of Advanced Atherosclerosis in Elderly Women," *Calcified Tissue International* 73, no. 1 (July 2003): 15–20; S. G. Rostand, "Ultraviolet Light May Contribute to Geographic and Racial Blood Pressure Differences," *Hypertension* 30, no. 2 pt. 1 (1997): 150–56; R. Krause, M. Buhring, W. Hopfenmuller, M. F. Holick, and A. M. Sharma, "Ultraviolet B and Blood Pressure," *Lancet* 352, no. 9129 (1998): 709–10; M. Pfeifer, B. Begerow, H. W. Minne, D. Nachtigall, and C. Hansen, "Effects of a Short-Term Vitamin D3 and Calcium Supplementation on Blood Pressure and Parathyroid Hormone Levels in Elderly Women," *Journal Clinical Endocrinology Metabolism* 86, no. 4 (2001): 1633–37; *Annals of the New York Academy of Sciences* (1999): 107–19. P. E. Normal and J. T. Powell, "Vitamin D, Shedding Light on the Development of Disease in Peripheral Arteries," *Arteriosclerosis, Thrombosis, and Vascular Biology* 25 (2005): 39.

CHAPTER SIX

1. S. Park and M. A. Johnson, "Living in Low-Latitude Regions in the United States Does Not Prevent Poor Vitamin D Status," *Nutrition Reviews* 63, no. 6 pt. 1 (June 2005): 203–209.

2. N. J. Shaw and B. R. Pal, "Vitamin D Deficiency in UK Asian Families: Activating a New Concern," *Archives of Disease in Childhood* 86, no. 3 (March 2002): 147–50.

3. M. M. Salamolun, A. S. Kizirian, R. I. Tannous, M. M. Nabulsi, M. K. Choucair, M. E. Deeb, and G. A. El-Haff Fuleihan, "Low Calcium and Vitamin D Intake in Healthy Children and Adolescents and Their Correlates," *European Journal of Clinical Nutrition* (October 6, 2004).

4. Saleh H. Sedrani, Abdel Wahab T. H. Elidrissy, and Kamal M. El Arabi, "Sunlight and Vitamin D Status in Normal Saudi Subjects," *American Journal of Clinical Nutrition* 38 (July 1983): 129–32; Mona S. Calvo, Susan J. Whiting, and Curtis N. Barton, "Vitamin D Intake: A Global Perspective of Current Status," *Journal of Nutrition* 135, no. 2 (February 2005): 310–17.

5. Alok Sachan, Renu Gupta, Vinita Das, Anjoo Agarwal, Pradeep K. Awasthi, and Vijayalakshmi Bhatia, "High Prevalence of Vitamin D Deficiency among Pregnant Women and Their Newborns in Northern India," *American Journal of Clinical Nutrition* 81, no. 5 (May 2005): 1060–64.

6. Sedrani et al., "Sunlight and Vitamin D Status in Normal Saudi Subjects."

7. Erika Friedl, *Women of Deh Koh: Lives in an Iranian Village* (New York: Penguin, 1989), pp. 26–46.

8. Theobald A. Palm, "The Geographical Distribution and Aetiology of Rickets," *Practitioner* (October 1890): 270–79; (November 1890): 321–42.

9. Pearl S. Buck, *The Good Earth* (New York: Washington Square Press, 1931); Ida Pruitt, *A Daughter of Han: The Autobiography of a Chinese Working Woman* (Stanford, CA : Stanford University Press, 1967), p. 22.

10. Patricia Buckley Ebrey, *The Inner Quarters: Marriage and the Lives of Chinese Women in the Sung Period* (Berkeley: University of California Press, 1993), p. 175.

11. J. P. Neilson, T. Lavender, S. Quenby, and S. Wray, "Obstructed Labour," *British Medical Bulletin* 67 (2003): 191–204.

12. Ibid.

13. "Cesarean Section: A Brief History," National Library of Medicine, http://www.nlm.nih.gov/hmd/pdf/cesarean.pdf (accessed November 20, 2008).

14. John Duffy, ed., *History of Medicine in Louisiana*, vol. 2 (Baton Rouge: Louisiana State University Press, 1962), p. 74.

15. J. Marion Sims, "Further Observations on Trismus Nascentium with Cases Illustrating Its Etiology and Treatment," *American Journal of the Medical Sciences* 16 (July 1848): 59–79; J. Marion Sims, *The Story of My Life*, ed. H. Marion Sims (New York: D. Appleton, 1886); Deborah Kuhn McGregor, *From Midwives to Medicine: The Birth of American Gynecology* (New Brunswick, NJ: Rutgers University Press, 1998).

16. McGregor, *From Midwives to Medicine*, p. 40; Duffy, *History of Medicine in Louisiana*, p. 74.

17. Duffy, *History of Medicine in Louisiana*, p. 68.

18. Justin C. Konje and Oladapo A. Ladipo, "Nutrition and Obstructed Labor." *American Journal of Clinical Nutrition* 72, suppl. (2000): 291S–97S.

19. Neilson et al., "Obstructed Labour"; Konje and Ladipo, "Nutrition and Obstructed Labor."

20. "Preliminary Births for 2004: Infant and Maternal Health" National Center for Health Statistics, Centers for Disease Control, US Department of Health and Human Services, www.cdc.gov/nchs/products/pubs/pubd/hestats/prelimbirths04; M. Khawaja, R. Jurdi, and T. Kabakian-Khasholian, "Rising Trends in Cesarean Section Rates in Egypt," *Birth* 31, no. 1 (March 31, 2004): 12–16; Iliana R. Chertook, Ilana Shoham-Vardi, and Hallek Mordechai, "Four-Month Breastfeeding Duration in Postcesarean Women of Different Cultures in the Israeli Negev," *Journal of Perinatal and Neonatal Nursing* 18, no. 2 (April/June 2004): 145–61.

21. P. H. Shiono, D. McNellis, and G. G. Rhoads, "Reasons for the Rising Cesarean Delivery Rates: 1978–1984," *Obstetrics and Gynecology* 69, no. 5 (May 1987): 696–700; See CDC report, http://www.cdc.gov/nchs/releases/03news/lowbirth.htm.

22. Shiono et al., "Reasons for the Rising Cesarean Delivery Rates: 1978–1984."

23. Iraj Forouzan and Mabel M. Bonilla, "Dystocia," *E-Medicine*, http://www.emedicine.com/med/topic3280.htm. (accessed December 23, 2004).

24. Rae Davies, "CIMS Alarmed by Highest U.S. Cesarean Rate Ever," http://www.vbac.com/hottopic/highestrate.html.

25. "Cost Considerations," Novatrix Medical Corporation, http://www.bekker-studios.com/novatrix/costconsiderations.html; "Rates of Cesarean Delivery: United States, 1991," Office of Vital and Health Statistics Systems, National Center for Health Statistics, Centers for Disease Control, http://www.cdc.gov/mmwr/preview/mmwrhtml/00020285.htm.

26. Denise Grady, "After Caesareans, Some See Higher Insurance Cost," *New York Times*, http://www.nytimes.com/2008/06/01/health/01insure.html?_r=1 (accessed October 13, 2008).

27. Justin C. Konje and Oladapo A. Ladipo, "Nutrition and Obstructed Labor." G. K. Oyakhire, "Environmental Factors Influencing Maternal Mortality in Zaria, Nigeria," *Rural Sociology Health Journal* 100, no. 2 (April 1980): 72–74; L. Ar. Airede and B. A. Ekele, "Adolescent Maternal Mortality in Sokoto, Nigeria," *Journal of Obstetrics and Gynaecology* 23, no. 2 (March 2003): 163–65.

28. Kenneth Bjorklund, "Minimally Invasive Surgery for Obstructed Labor: A Review of Symphysiotomy during the Twentieth Century (Including 5,000 Cases)," *BJOG: International Journal of Obstetrics and Gynecology* 109 (March 2002): 236–48.

29. "Symphysiotomy," *Managing Complications in Pregnancy and Childbirth: A Guide for Midwives and Doctors*, Department of Reproductive Health and Research, World Health Organization, 2002, http://www.who.int/reproductive-health/impac/Procedures/Symphysiotomy.

30. Bjorklund, "Minimally Invasive Surgery for Obstructed Labor."

31. Konje and Ladipo, "Nutrition and Obstructed Labor"; C. P. Shirima and J. L. Kinabo, "Nutritional Status and Birth Outcomes of Adolescent Pregnant Girls in Morogoro, Coast, and Dar es Salaam Regions, Tanzania," *Nutrition* 21, no. 1 (January 2005): 32–38.

32. P. Garner, M. S. Kramer, and I. Chalmers, "Might Efforts to Increase Birthweight in Undernourished Women Do More Harm Than Good?" *Lancet* 340, no. 8826 (October 24, 1999): 1021–23; Konje and Ladipo. "Nutrition and Obstructed Labor"; Mtimavalye, van der Does, and Maathuis, "The Relationship between Increasing Birthweight and Cephalopelvic Disproportion in Dar Es Salaam, Tanzania," *Journal of Obstetrics and Gynaecology of the British Commonwealth* 81, no. 5 (May 1974): 380–82; L. Brunvand, S. S. Shah, S. Bergstrom, and E. Haug, "Vitamin D Deficiency in Pregnancy Is Not Associated with Obstructed Labor. A Study among Pakistani Women in Karachi," *Acta Obstetricia et Gynecologica Scandinavica* 77, no. 3 (March 1998): 303–306.

33. George Constable, *The Neanderthals*, Emergence of Man series (New York: Time-Life Books, 1973), p. 15.

34. Ibid.

35. Douglas Palmer, "Big Chill Killed Off the Neanderthals," *New Scientist* (January 24, 2004): 10–11.

36. "Portrait of a Neanderthal," *New Scientist* (July 24, 2004): 17.

37. Ezra Zubrow, "The Demographic Modeling of Neanderthal Extinction," in *The Human Revolution: Behavioural and Biological Perspectives on the Origin of Modern Humans* vol. 1, ed. P. Mellars and C. B. Stringer (Edinburgh: Edinburgh University Press), pp. 212–31.

38. Constable, *The Neanderthals*.

39. Paul Graves, "New Models and Metaphors for the Neanderthal Debate," *Current Anthropology* 32, no. 5 (December 1991): 533.

40. James C. Chatters, *Ancient Encounters: Kennewick Man and the First Americans* (New York: Simon & Schuster, 2001), p. 213.

41. Reinhold Vieth, "Effects of Vitamin D on Bone and Natural Selection of Skin Color: How Much Vitamin D Nutrition Are We Talking About?" *Bone Loss and Osteoporosis: An Anthropological Perspective*, ed. Sabrina C. Agarwal and Sam D. Stout (New York: Kluwer Academic/Plenum Publishers, 2003), p. 148.

42. Sheila F. Mahoney and Lorraine Halinka Malcoe, "Cesarean Delivery in Native American Women: Are Low Rates Explained by Practices Common to the Indian Health Service?" *Birth* 32, no. 3 (September 2005): 170–78; J. Hallfrisch, C. Veillon, K. Y. Patterson, A. D. Hill, I. Benn, B. Holiday, R. Burns, S. Zhonnie, F. Price, and A. Sorenson, "Bone-Related Mineral Content of Water Samples Collected on the Navajo Reservation," *Toxicology* 149 nos. 2–3 (August 21, 2000): 143–48.

43. Judith G. Hallfrisch, "Boning Up on Navajo Food Habits," *Agricultural Research* (June 2001).

44. Chun-Yuh Yang, Hui-Fen Chiu, Chi-Ching Chang, Trong-Neng Wu, and Fung Chang Sung, "Association of Very Low Birth Weight with Calcium Levels in Drinking Water," *Environmental Research* 89 (2002): 189–94; S. Roux, C. Baudoin, D. Boute, M. Brazier, V. De La Gueronniere, and M. C. De Vernejoul, "Biological Effects of Drinking-Water Mineral Composition on Calcium Balance and Bone Remodeling Markers," *Journal of Nutrition, Health & Aging* 8, no. 5 (2004): 380–84; Philippe Garzon and Mark J. Eisenberg, "Variation in the Mineral Content of Commercially Available Bottled Waters: Implications for Health and Disease," *American Journal of Medicine* 105 (August 1998): 125–30; I. Aptel, A. Cance-Rouzaud, and H. Grandjean, "Association between Calcium Ingested from Drinking Water and Femoral Bone Density in Elderly Women: Evidence from the EPIDOS Cohort," *Journal of Bone and Mineral Research* 14, no. 5 (May 1999): 829–33.

CHAPTER SEVEN

1. D. Kunz, "Chronobiotic Protocol and Circadian Sleep Propensity Index: New Tools for Clinical Routine and Research on Melatonin and Sleep," *Pharmacopsychiatry* 37, no. 4 (July 2004): 139–46.

2. Tamara Pringsheim, "Cluster Headache: Evidence for a Disorder of Circadian Rhythm and Hypothalamic Function," *Canadian Journal of Neurological Sciences* 29, no. 1 (February 2002): 33–40.

3. M. M. Macchi and J. N. Bruce, "Human Pineal Physiology and Functional Significance of Melatonin," *Frontiers in Neuroendocrinology* 25, nos. 3–4 (September/December 2004): 177–95.

4. Russell G. Foster and Leon Kreitzman, *Rhythms of Life: The Biological Clocks That Control the Daily Lives of Every Living Thing* (New Haven, CT: Yale University Press, 2004), p. 96.

5. A. J. Lewy, T. A. Wehr, F. K. Goodwin, D. A. Newsome, and S. P, Markey, "Light Suppresses Melatonin Secretion in Humans," *Science* 210, no. 4475 (December 12, 1980): 1267–69.

6. John N. Ott, *Health and Light: The Effects of Natural and Artificial Light on Man and Other Living Things* (Greenwich, CN: Devin-Adair Co., 1973), pp. 37–39.

7. Ibid.

8. Ibid.

9. "Health Effects of Overexposure to the Sun," SunWise Program, US Environmental Protection Agency, http://www.epa.gov/SUNWISE/uvandhealth.html (accessed October 13, 2008).

10. Foster and Kreitzman, *Rhythms of Life*, p. 202. Masako Kobayashi and Maiko

Kobayashi, "The Relationship between Obesity and Seasonal Variation in Body Weight among Elementary School Children in Tokyo," *Economics and Human Biology* 4, no. 2 (June 2006): 253–61.

11. Jeffrey S. Flier, Mark Harris, and Anthony N. Hollenberg, "Leptin, Nutrition, and the Thyroid: The Why, the Wherefore, and the Wiring," *Journal of Clinical Investigation* 105, no. 7 (April 2000): 859–61.

12. C. L. Adam and J. G. Mercer, "Appetite Regulation and Seasonality: Implications for Obesity," *Proceedings of the Nutrition Society* 63, no. 3 (Auguat 2004): 413–19; Farid F. Chehab, Jun Qiu, and Scott Ogus, "The Use of Animal Models to Dissect the Biology of Leptin," *Recent Progress in Hormone Research* 59 (2004): 245–66.

13. V. Matkovic, J. Z. Ilich, N. E. Badenhop, M. Skugor, A. Clairmont, D. Klisovic, and J. D. Landoll, "Gain in Body Fat Is Inversely Related to the Nocturnal Rise in Serum Leptin Level in Young Females," *Journal of Clinical Endocrinology and Metabolism* 82, no. 5 (1997): 1368–72; Flier, Harris, and Hollenberg, "Leptin, Nutrition, and the Thyroid."

14. Mayer Hillman and Jon Parker, "Communications: More Daylight, Less Electricity," *Energy Policy* 16, no. 5 (October 1988): 514–15.

15. Geoffry McEnany and Kathryn A. Lee, "Owls, Larks and the Significance of Morningness/Eveningness Rhythm Propensity in Psychiatric-Mental Health Nursing," *Issues in Mental Health Nursing* 21, no. 2 (March 1, 2000): 203–16.

16. Susan A. Ferguson, David F. Preusser, Adrian K. Lund, Paul L. Zador, and Robert G. Ulmer, "Daylight Saving Time and Motor Vehicle Crashes: The Reduction in Pedestrian and Vehicle Occupant Fatalities," *American Journal of Public Health* 85, no. 1 (January 1995): 92–96; G. J. Hicks, J. W. Davis, and R. A. Hicks, "Fatal Alcohol-Related Traffic Crashes Increase Subsequent to Changes to and from Daylight Savings Time," *Perceptual Motor Skills* 86, no. 3 pt. 1 (June 1998): 879–82.

17. Tamara Pringsheim, "Cluster Headache: Evidence for a Disorder of Circadian Rhythm and Hypothalamic Function," *Canadian Journal of Neurological Sciences* 29 (2002): 33–40.

18. A. T. Landsdowne and S. C. Provost, "Vitamin D3 Enhances Mood in Healthy Subjects during Winter," *Psychopharmacology* 135, no. 4 (February 1998): 319–23.

19. S. J. Crowley, C. Lee, C. Y. Tseng, L. F. Fogg, and C. I. Eastman, "Combinations of Bright Light, Scheduled Dark, Sunglasses, and Melatonin to Facilitate Circadian Entrainment to Night Shift Work," *Journal of Biological Rhythms* 18, no. 6 (December 2003): 513–23.

20. Norman E. Rosenthal, *Winter Blues: Seasonal Affective Disorder, What It Is and How to Overcome It* (New York: Guilford Press, 1998), p. 102; D. H. Avery, D. N. Eder, M. A. Bolte, C. J. Hellekson, D. L. Dunner, M. V. Vitiello, and P. N. Prinz, "Dawn Simulation and Bright Light in the Treatment of SAD: A Controlled Study," *Biological Psychiatry* 50, no. 3 (August 1, 2001): 205–26.

21. Avery et al., "Dawn Simulation and Bright Light in the Treatment of SAD."

22. V. Srinivasan et al., "Therapeutic Actions of Melatonin in Cancer: Possible Mecanisms," *Integrative Cancer Therapies* 7, no. 3 (September 2008): 189–203; F. M. Gloth III, W. Alam, and B. Hollis, "Vitamin D vs. Broad Spectrum Phototherapy in the Treatment of Seasonal Affective Disorder," *Journal of Nutritional Health and Aging* 3, no. 1 (1999): 5–7.

23. Foster and Kreitzman, *Rhythms of Life*, p. 210; Macchi and Bruce, "Human Pineal Physiology and Functional Significance of Melatonin."

24. Foster and Kreitzman, *Rhythms of Life*; N. Buscemi, B. Vanermeer, R. Pandya, N. Hooton, L. Tjosvold, L. Harling, G. Baker, S. Vohra, and T. Klassen, "Melatonin for Sleep Disorders," Evidence Report/Technology Assessment 108 AHRQ pub. no. 05-E002-1 (November 2004); H. Olders, "Average Sunrise Time Predicts Depression Prevalence," *Journal of Psychosomatic Research* 55, no. 2 (August 2003): 999–1005.

25. Nic Fleming, "Summer Lends a Helping Hand," *(London) Daily Telegraph*, October 18, 2005, p. 10.

26. "Low Melatonin Associated with Increased Risk of Breast Cancer in Postmenopausal Women," *Science Daily, Journal of the National Cancer Institute* (June 16, 2008), http://www.sciencedaily.com/releases/2008/06/080610161255.htm (accessed August 5, 2008).

27. "New Research Shows Artificial Light at Night Stimulates Breast Cancer Growth in Laboratory Mice," NIH press release, December 19, 2005, www.webwire.com.

28. Richard G. Stevens, "Artificial Lighting in the Industrialized World: Circadian Disruption and Breast Cancer," *Cancer Causes and Control* 17, no. 4 (May 2006): 501–507.

29. R. J. Reiter et al., "Light at Night, Chronodisruption, Melatonin Suppression, and Cancer Risk: A Review," *Critical Reviews in Oncogenesis* 13, no. 4 (2007): 303–28.

30. L. Edwards and P. Torcellini. "A Literature Review of the Effects of Natural Light on Building Occupants," technical report NREL/TP-550-30769 National Renewable Energy Laboratory (July 2002), p. 3. See http:://ornl.gov/sci/solar/NREL _TP_550_30769.pdf (accessed October 16, 2008).

31. Ibid.; L. W. Mayron, J. Ott, R. Nations, and E. L. Mayron, "Light, Radiation, and Academic Behavior," *Academic Therapy* 10, no. 1 (1974): 33–47.

32. Edwards and Torcellini, "A Literature Review of the Effects of Natural Light on Building Occupants."

33. Ibid., p. 18.

34. Ibid., p. 19.

35. Kenneth J. Cooper, "Study Says Natural Classroom Lighting Can Aid Achievement," *Washington Post*, November 26, 1999, p. A-14.

36. "Daylighting," Neuro-Learning Systems, www.neurolearning.net/Daylighting.htm (accessed October 16, 2008).

37. Edwards and Torcellini, "A Literature Review of the Effects of Natural Light on Building Occupants, " p. 32.

CHAPTER EIGHT

1. Kenneth Chang, "Globe Grows Darker as Sunshine Diminishes 10% to 37%," *New York Times*, May 13 2004, http://www.commondreams.org/headlines04/0513-01.htm (accessed October 16, 2008).

2. "Global Dimming," broadcast on the BBC program *Science and Nature*, January 15, 2005, www.bbc.co.uk/sn/tvradio/programmes/horizon/dimming_transcript; Martin Wild, Hans Gilgen, Andreas Roesch, Atsumu Ohmura, Charles N. Long, Ellsworth G. Dutton, Bruce Forgan, Ain Kallis, Viivi Russak, and Anatoly Tsvetkov, "From Dimming to Brightening: Decadal Changes in Solar Radiation at Earth's Surface," *Science* 308, no. 5723 (May 6, 2005): 847–50.

3. Beate G. Liepert, "Observed Reductions of Surface Solar Radiation at Sites in the United States and Worldwide from 1961 to 1990," *Geophysical Research Letters* (April 2002); Chang, "Globe Grows Darker as Sunshine Diminishes 10% to 37%."

4. M. L. Roderick and G. D. Farquahar, "Changes in Australian Pan Evaporation from 1970 to 2002," *International Journal of Climatology* 24, no. 9 (July 2004): 1077–90.

5. "Global Dimming," *Science and Nature*.

6. "Some African Drought Linked to Warmer Indian Ocean, NASA Data Show," *Science Daily*, August 7, 2008, http://www.sciencedaily.com/releases/2008/08/080805124005.htm (accessed October 17, 2008).

7. R. A. C. Mitchell, C. L. Gibbard, F. J. Mitchell, and D. W. Lawlor, "Effects of Shading in Different Developmental Phases on Biomass and Grain Yield of Winter Wheat at Ambient and Elevated CO2," *Plant Cell and Environment* 19, no. 5 (1996): 615–21; Simon L. Lewis, Yadvinder Malhi, and Oliver L. Phillips, "Fingerprinting the Impacts of Global Change on Tropical Forests," *Philosophical Transactions: Biological Sciences* 359, no. 1443 (March 29, 2004): 437–62; S. L. Lewis, O. L. Phillips, T. R. Baker, et al., "Concerted Changes in Tropical Forest Structure and Dynamids: Evidence from 50 South American Long-Term Plots," *Philosophical Transactions: Biological Sciences* 359, no. 1443 (March 2004): 421–36.

8. Maximilian Auffhammer, V. Ramanathan, and Jeffrey R. Vincent, "Integrated Model Shows That Atmospheric Brown Clouds and Greenhouse Gases Have Reduced Rice Harvests in India," *Proceedings of National Academy of Sciences* 103, no. 52 (December 26, 2006): 19668–72.

9. Ibid., p. 19670.

10. Dale W. Griffin, Virginia H. Garrison, Jay R. Herman, and Eugene A. Shinn,

"African Desert Dust in the Caribbean Atmosphere: Microbiology and Public Health," *Aerobiologia* 17 (2001): 203–13; Doug Struck, "Dust Storms Overseas Carry Contaminants to U. S.," *Washington Post*, February 6, 2008, http://www.washingtonpost.com/wp-dyn/content/article/2008/02/05/AR2008020502950_pf.html (accessed October 18, 2008).

11. Dale W. Griffin and Christina A. Kellogg, "Dust Storms and Their Impact on Ocean and Human Health: Dust in Earth's Atmosphere," *EcoHealth* 1 (July 13, 2004): 284–95; Struck, "Dust Storms Overseas Carry Contaminants to U. S."

12. Bryan Walsh, "Beijing Smog Cleanup: Has It Worked?" *Time*, August 15, 2008, http://www.time.com/time/health/article/0,8599,1833371,00.htm (accessed October 18, 2008); Jon Hamilton, "Pollution Found to Inhibit Rainfall in China," NPR, March 8, 2007, http://www.npr.org/templates/story/story.php?storyId=7779885. There are several programs on the NPR Web site describing how the anomaly of polluted clouds can actually prevent rainfall.

13. Struck, "Dust Storms Overseas Carry Contaminants to U. S."

14. Ibid.

15. Griffin and Kellogg, "Dust Storms and Their Impact on Ocean and Human Health."

16. Bjorn Carey, "Bacteria & Fungi Ride Dust across Oceans," *LiveScience*, June 5, 2006, http://www.livescience.com/environment/060605_disease_dust.html (accessed October 3, 2008). Griffin and Kellogg, "Dust Storms and Their Impact on Ocean and Human Health," p. 291.

17. Dale W. Griffin, "Atmospheric Movement of Microorganisms in Clouds of Desert Dust and Implications for Human Health," *Clinical Microbiology Reviews* 20, no. 3 (July 2007): 459–77.

18. Carey, "Bacteria & Fungi Ride Dust across Oceans."

19. Griffin, "Atmospheric Movement of Microorganisms in Clouds of Desert Dust and Implications for Human Health."

20. Struck, "Dust Storms Overseas Carry Contaminants to U. S."

21. Ibid.

22. Griffin, "Atmospheric Movement of Microorganisms in Clouds of Desert Dust and Implications for Human Health."

BIBLIOGRAPHY

Abbot, Charles Greeley. *The Sun and the Welfare of Man*. New York: Smithsonian Institution Series, 1929.

Adam, C. L., and J. G. Mercer. "Appetite Regulation and Seasonality: Implications for Obesity." *Proceedings of the Nutrition Society* 263, no. 3 (August 2004): 413–19.

Affleck, Paul. "Sun Exposure and Health." *Nursing Standard* 19, no. 47 (August 3–9, 2005): 50–55.

Airede, L. A., and B. A. Ekele. "Adolescent Maternal Mortality in Sokoto, Nigeria." *Journal of Obstetrics and Gynaecology* 23, no. 2 (March 2003): 163–65.

Alcott, Louisa May. *Hospital Sketches*. Edited by Alice Fahs. Boston: Bedford/St. Martin's, 2004.

Allen, Scott. "BU Advocate of Sunlight Draws Ire." *Boston Globe*, April 13, 2004, A1.

Apple, Rima D. "Patenting University Research." *ISIS* 80 (1989): 374–94.

———. *Vitamania: Vitamins in American Culture*. New Brunswick, NJ: Rutgers University Press, 1996.

Aptel, I., A. Cance-Rouzaud, and H. Grandjean. "Association between Calcium Ingested from Drinking Water and Femoral Bone Density in Elderly Women: Evidence from the EPIDOS Cohort." *Journal of Bone and Mineral Research* 14, no. 5 (May 1999): 829–33.

Arunabh, S., S. Pollack, J. Yeh, and J. F. Aloia. "Body Fat Content and 25-Hydroxyvitamin D Levels in Healthy Women." *Journal of Clinical Endocrinology and Metabolism* 88, no. 1 (January 2003): 157–61.

Auffhammer, Maximilian, V. Ramanathan, and Jeffrey R. Vincent. "Integrated Model Shows That Atmospheric Brown Clouds and Greenhouse Gases Have Reduced Rice Harvests in India." *Proceedings of National Academy of Sciences* 103, no. 52 (December 26, 2006): 19668–72.

Avery, D. H., D. N. Eder, M. A. Bolte, C. J. Hellekson, D. L. Dunner, M. V. Vitiello, and P. N. Prinz. "Dawn Simulation and Bright Light in the Treatment of SAD: A Controlled Study." *Biological Psychiatry* 50, no. 3 (August 1, 2001): 205–26.

Balch, James F., and Phyllis A. Balch. *Prescription for Nutritional Healing*. Garden City, NY: Avery Publishing, 1997.

Becker, Axel, Darryl W. Eyles, John J. McGrath, and Gisela Grecksch. "Transient Prenatal Vitamin D Deficiency Is Associated with Subtle Alternations in Learning and Memory Functions in Adult Rats." *Behavioural Brain Research* 161, no. 2 (June 20, 2005): 306–12.

Berwick, Marianne, Bruce K. Armstrong, Leah Ben-Porat, et al. "Sun Exposure and

Mortality from Melanoma." *Journal of the National Cancer Institute* 97, no. 3 (February 2, 2005): 195–99.

Best, C. H., and E. W. McHenry. "The Vitamins." *Canadian Medical Association Journal* (April 1930): 540–45.

"Biochemistry and Physiology of Vitamin D." Vitamin D Home Page. University of California-Riverside. http://vitamind.ucr.edu/biochem.html (accessed October 17, 2008).

Bischoff-Ferrari, H. A., W. C. Willett, J. B. Wong, E. Giovannucci, T. Dietrich, and B. Dawson-Hughes. "Fracture Prevention with Vitamin D Supplementation: A Meta-analysis of Randomized Controlled Trials." *Journal of the American Medical Association* 293, no. 18 (May 2005): 2257–64.

Bjorklund, Kenneth. "Minimally Invasive Surgery for Obstructed Labor: A Review of Symphysiotomy during the Twentieth Century (Including 5,000 Cases)." *BJOG: International Journal of Obstetrics and Gynaecology* 109 (March 2002): 236–48.

Blois, Marsden S. "Vitamin D, Sunlight, and Natural Selection." *Science* 159 (1968): 652–53.

Blunt, Katharine, and Ruth Cowan. *Ultraviolet Light and Vitamin D in Nutrition.* Chicago: University of Chicago Press, 1930.

Bodiwala, D., C. J. Luscombe, M. E. French, et al. "Susceptibility to Prostate Cancer: Studies on Interactions between UVR Exposure and Skin Type." *Carcinogenesis* 24, no. 4 (April 1, 2003): 711–17.

Bowyer, S. L., and J. R. Hollister. "Limb Pain in Childhood." *Pediatric Clinics of North America* 31, no. 5 (October 1984): 1053–81.

Boyles, Salynn. "Calcium + Vitamin D = Lower Cancer Risk." *WebMD.* http://mywebmd.com/contentArticle/77/95547.htm (accessed November 18, 2007).

Brown, A. J., C. S. Ritter, L. S. Holliday, J. C. Knutson, and S. A. Strugnell. "Tissue Distribution and Activity Studies of 1,24-Dihydroxyvitamin D2, a Metabolite of Vitamin D2 with Low Calcemic Activity in Vivo." *Biochemistry Pharmacology* 68, no. 7 (October 1, 2004): 1289–96.

Brown, A. S., and E. S. Susser. "Prenatal Nutritional Deficiency and Risk of Adult Schizophrenia." *Schizophrenia Bulletin* 34, no. 6 (August 4, 2008).

Brunvand, L., S. S. Shah, S. Bergstrom, and E. Haug. "Vitamin D Deficiency in Pregnancy Is Not Associated with Obstructed Labor; A Study among Pakistani Women in Karachi." *Acta. Obstetrics and Gynecology Scandinavia* 77, no. 3 (March 1998): 303–306.

Brustad, M., T. Sandanger, L. Aksnes, and E. Lund. "Vitamin D Status in a Rural Population of Northern Norway with High Fish Liver Consumption." *Public Health Nutrition* 7, no. 6 (September 2004): 783–89.

Buck, Pearl S. *The Good Earth.* New York: Washington Square Press, 1931.

Buscemi, N., B. Vanermeer, R. Pandya, N. Hooton, L. Tjosvold, L. Harling, G. Baker, S. Vohra, and T. Klassen. "Melatonin for Sleep Disorders." Evidence report/technology assessment 108 AHRQ pub. no. 05-E002-1 (November 2004).

Calabro, J. J., A. E. Wachtel, W. B. Holgerson, and M. M. Repice. "Growing Pains: Fact or Fiction?" *Postgraduate Medicine* 59, no. 2 (February 1976): 66–72.

"'Calcium Crisis' Affects American Youth." National Institutes of Health, December 10, 2001. http://www.nichd.nih.gov/new/releases/calcium_crisis.cfm?from=milk (accessed October 16, 2008).

Calvo, Mona S., and Susan J. Whiting. "Overview of the Proceedings from Experimental Biology 2004 Symposium: Vitamin D Insufficiency: A Significant Risk Factor in Chronic Disease and Potential Disease-Specific Biomarkers of Vitamin D Sufficiency." *Journal of Nutrition* 135, no. 2 (February 2005): 301–303.

Calvo, Mona S., Susan J. Whiting, and Curtis N. Barton. "Vitamin D Fortification in the United States and Canada: Current Status and Data Needs." *American Journal of Clinical Nutrition* 80, suppl. (December 2004): 1710S–16S.

———. "Vitamin D Intake: A Global Perspective of Current Status." *Journal of Nutrition* 135, no. 2 (February 2005): 310–17.

Campbell, Joseph. *The Hero with a Thousand Faces*. Princeton, NJ: Princeton University Press, 1949.

Cannell, J. J., R. Vieth, J. C. Umhau, M. F. Holick, W. B. Grant, S. Madronich, C. F. Garland, and E. Giovannucci. "Epidemic Influenza and Vitamin D," *Epidemiology and Infection* 134, no. 6 (December 2006): 1129–40.

Cannell, John. "Autism and Vitamin D." *Medical Hypotheses* (October 4, 2007).

———. *Vitamin D Newsletter*. Vitamin D Council (July 2008).

Carey, Bjorn. "Bacteria & Fungi Ride Dust across Oceans." *LiveScience*, June 5, 2006. http://www.livescience.com/environment/060605_disease_dust.html (accessed October 3, 2008).

Carlson, Laurie Winn. *William J. Spillman and the Birth of Agricultural Economics*. Columbia: University of Missouri Press, 2005.

"Cesarean Section: A Brief History." National Library of Medicine, National Institutes of Health. http://www.nlm.nih.gov/exhibition/cesarean/index.html (accessed October 18, 2008).

Chang, Kenneth. "Globe Grows Darker as Sunshine Diminishes 10% to 37%." *New York Times*, May 13, 2004. http://www.commondreams.org/headlines04/0513-01.htm (accessed October 18, 2008).

Chatters, James C. *Ancient Encounters: Kennewick Man and the First Americans*. New York: Simon & Schuster, 2001.

Chee, W. S. S., A. R. Suriah, S. P. Chan, Y. Zaitun, and Y. M. Chan. "The Effect of Milk Supplementation on Bone Mineral Density in Postmenopausal Chinese Women in Malasia." *Osteoporosis International* 14 (2003): 828–34.

Chehab, Farid F., Jun Qiu, and Scott Ogus. "The Use of Animal Models to Dissect the Biology of Leptin." *Recent Progress in Hormone Research* 59 (2004): 245–66.

Chen, T. C., and M. F. Holick. "Vitamin D and Prostate Cancer Prevention and Treatment." *Trends in Endocrinology and Metabolism* 14, no. 9 (Nov 2003): 423–30.

Chen, T. C., A. Shao, H. Heath III, and M. F. Holick. "An Update on the Vitamin D Content of Fortified Milk from the United States and Canada." *New England Journal of Medicine* 329 (1993): 1507.

Chertook, Iliana R., Ilana Shoham-Vardi, and Hallek Mordechai. "Four-Month Breastfeeding Duration in Postcesarean Women of Different Cultures in the Israeli Negev." *Journal of Perinatal and Neonatal Nursing* 18, no. 2 (April/June 2004): 145–61.

Chesney, Russell. "Rickets: The Third Wave." *Clinical Pediatrics* (April 2002).

Chiricone, D., N. G. De Santo, and M. Cirillo. "Unusual Cases of Chronic Intoxication by Vitamin D." *Journal of Nephrology* 16, no. 6 (November/December 2003): 917–21.

Cho, E., S. A. Smith-Warner, D. Spiegelman, et al. "Dairy Foods, Calcium, and Colorectal Cancer: A Pooled Analysis of 10 Cohort Studies." *Journal of the National Cancer Institute* 96, no. 13 (July 1996): 1015–22.

Clark, Janet Howell. *Lighting in Relation to Public Health.* Baltimore: Williams and Wilkins Co., 1924.

Constable, George. *The Neanderthals.* Emergence of Man series. New York: Time-Life Books, 1973.

Cooper, Kenneth J. "Study Says Natural Classroom Lighting Can Aid Achievement," *Washington Post*, November 26, 1999, A-14.

"Cost Considerations." Novatrix Medical Corporation. http://www.bekker-studios .com/novatrix/costconsiderations.html (accessed November 2, 2007).

Cramer, Frederick H. *Astrology in Roman Law and Politics.* Philadelphia: American Philosophical Society, 1954.

Crocombe, S., M. Z. Mughal, and J. L. Berry. "Symptomatic Vitamin D Deficiency Among Non-Caucasian Adolescents Living in the United Kingdom." *Archives of Disease in Childhood* 89, no. 2 (February 2004): 197–99.

Crowley, S. J., C. Lee, C. Y. Tseng, L. F. Fogg, and C. I. Eastman. "Combinations of Bright Light, Scheduled Dark, Sunglasses, and Melatonin to Facilitate Circadian Entrainment to Night Shift Work." *Journal of Biological Rhythms* 18, no. 6 (December 2003): 513–23.

Cruse, L. M., J. Valeriano, F. B. Vasey, and J. D. Carter. "Prevalence of Evaluation and Treatment of Glucocorticoid-Induced Osteoporosis in Men." *Journal of Clinical Rheumatology* 12, no. 5 (October 2006): 221–25.

Cumont, Franz. *The Mysteries of Mithra.* Translation by Thomas J. McCormack. New York: Dover Publications, 1956.

Davies, Rae. "CIMS Alarmed by Highest U.S. Cesarean Rate Ever." http://www.vbac
.com (accessed October 6, 2007).

Dawodu, A., and C. L. Wagner. "Mother-Child Vitamin D Deficiency: An International
Perspective." *Archives of Disease in Childhood* 92, no. 9 (September 1, 2007):
737–40.

Dawson-Hughes, B., G. E. Dallal, E. A. Krall, S. Harris, L. J. Sokoll, and G. Falconer. "Effect
of Vitamin D Supplementation on Wintertime and Overall Bone Loss in Healthy
Postmenopausal Women." *Annals of Internal Medicine* 115 (1991): 505–12.

Deftos, L. J., M. M. Miller, and D. W. Burton. "A High-Fat Diet Increases Calcitonin
Secretion in the Rat." *Bone and Mineral* 5, no. 3 (March 1989): 303–308.

De Kruif, Paul. *Men Against Death.* New York: Harcourt, Brace and Company, 1932.

DeLuca, Hector F. "Historical Overview." In *Vitamin D.*, 2nd ed, edited by D. Feldman,
F. H. Glorieux, and J. W. Pike. San Diego: Academic Press, 1997.

———. "Overview of General Physiologic Features and Functions of Vitamin D."
American Journal of Clinical Nutrition 80, no. 6 (December 2004): 1689S–96S.

———. "Vitamin D, the Vitamin and the Hormone." *Federation Proceedings* 33:
2211–2219 (1974).

"D-Ficiency." *Vegetarian Times* 322 (June 2004): 13.

Dhaval, Bodiwala, J. Lunscombe Christopher, Michael E. French, et al. "Susceptibility
to Prostate Cancer: Studies on Interactions between UVR Exposure and Skin
Type." *Carcinogenesis* 24, no. 4 (April 24, 2003): 711–17.

"Dietary Supplement Fact Sheet: Vitamin D." Office of Dietary Supplements. National
Institutes of Health. http://ods.od.nih.gov/factsheets/vitamind.asp (accessed
October 20, 2008).

Dixon, K. M., S. S. Deo, G. Wong, et al. "Skin Cancer Prevention: A Possible Role of
1,25-Dihydroxyvitamin D and Its Analogs." *Journal of Steroid Biochemistry and
Molecular Biology* 97, nos. 1–2 (October 2005): 137–43.

"Don't Be in the Dark about Tanning." *FDA Consumer Magazine.* US Food and Drug
Administration (November/December 2003). http://www.fda.gov/fdac/features/
2003/603_tan.html (accessed October 20, 2008).

Dubos, René. *Man Adapting.* New Haven, CT: Yale University Press, 1973.

Duffy, John, ed. *History of Medicine in Louisiana.* Vol. 2. Baton Rouge: Louisiana State
University Press, 1962.

Dukas, L., H. B. Staehelen, E. Schacht, and H. A. Bischoff. "Better Functional Mobility
in Community-Dwelling Elderly Is Related to D-Hormone Serum Levels and to
Daily Calcium Intake." *Journal of Nutrition Health and Aging* 9, no. 5 (Sep-
tember/October 2005): 347–51.

Dunn-Emke, S. R., G. Weidner, E. B. Peggengill, R. O. Marlin, C. Chi, and D. M.
Ornish. "Nutrient Adequacy of a Very Low-Fat Vegan Diet." *Journal of the American Dietetics Association* 105, no. 9 (September 2005): 1442–46.

East, B. "Mean Annual Hours of Sunshine and the Incidence of Dental Caries." *American Journal of Public Health* 29 (1939): 777–80.

Eberlein-Konig, B., T. Bergner, S. Diemer, and B. Przybill. "Evaluation of Phototoxic Properties of Some Food Additives: Sulfites Exhibit Prominent Phototoxicity." *Acta Dermato-Venereologica* 73, no. 5 (October 1993): 362–64.

Ebrey, Patricia Buckley. *The Inner Quarters: Marriage and the Lives of Chinese Women in the Sung Period.* Berkeley: University of California Press, 1993.

Edelson, R., C. Berger, F. Gasparro, et al. "Treatment of Cutaneous T-Cell Lymphoma by Extracorporeal Photochemotherapy. Preliminary Results." *New England Journal of Medicine* 316, no. 6 (February 5, 1987): 297–303.

Edwards, L., and P. Torcellini. "A Literature Review of the Effects of Natural Light on Building Occupants." Technical report NREL/TP-550-30769, National Renewable Energy Laboratory, July 2002.

Endo, I., and D. Inoue. "Effect of Calcium and Vitamin D on Skeletal Muscle." *Clinical Calcium* 13, no. 7 (July 2003): 905–907.

Enig, Mary G. *Know Your Fats: The Complete Primer for Understanding the Nutrition of Fats, Oils, and Cholesterol.* Silver Spring, MD: Bethesda Press, 2004.

Ensminger, Peter A. *Life under the Sun.* New Haven, CT: Yale University Press, 2001.

Etheridge, Elizabeth W. *The Butterfly Caste: A Social History of Pellagra in the South.* Westport, CT: Greenwood, 1972.

Evans, A. M., and S. D. Scutter. "Prevalence of 'Growing Pains' in Young Children." *Journal of Pediatrics* 145, no. 2 (August 2004): 255–58.

Eyles, Darryl, W. J. Brown, et al. "Vitamin D3 and Brain Development." *Neuroscience* 118, no. 3 (2003): 641–53.

Fagan, Brian. *The Long Summer: How Climate Changed Civilization.* New York: Basic Books, 2004.

Fears, T. R., C. C. Bird, D. Guerry, R. W. Sagebiel, M. H. Gail, D. E. Elder, A. Halpern, E. A. Holly, P. Hartge, and M. A. Tucker. "Average UVB Flux and TimeOutdoors Predict Melanoma Risk." *Cancer Research* 62, no. 14 (July 15, 2002): 3992–96.

Feldman, David, Francis H. Glorieux, and J. Wesley Pike, eds. *Vitamin D.* 2nd edition. San Diego: Academic Press, 1997.

Feldman, S. R., A. Liguori, M. Kucenic, S. R. Rapp, A. B. Fleischer, W. Lang, and M. Kaur. "Ultraviolet Exposure Is a Reinforcing Stimulus in Frequent Indoor Tanners." *Journal of the American Academy of Dermatology* 51, no. 1 (July 2004): 45–51.

Ferguson, Susan A., David F. Preusser, Adrian K. Lund, Paul L. Zador, and Robert G. Ulmer. "Daylight Saving Time and Motor Vehicle Crashes: The Reduction in Pedestrian and Vehicle Occupant Fatalities." *American Journal of Public Health* 85, no. 1 (January 1995): 92–96.

Feskanich, Diane, Jimg Ma, Charles S. Fuchs, et al. "Plasma Vitamin D Metabolites and

Risk of Colorectal Cancer in Women." *Cancer Epidemiology Biomarkers and Prevention* 13 (September 2004): 1502–1508.

Fildes, Valerie. *Wet Nursing: A History from Antiquity to the Present.* New York: Basil Blackwell, 1988.

Fleming, Nic. "Summer Lends a Helping Hand." *Daily Telegraph* (London), October 18, 2005, 10.

Flicker, L., R. Macinnis, M. Stein, S. Scherer, K. Mead, and C. Nowson. "Vitamin D to Prevent Falls in Older People in Residential Care." *Asia Pacific Journal of Clinical Nutrition* 14, suppl. (2005): S18.

Flier, Jeffrey S., Mark Harris, and Anthony N. Hollenberg. "Leptin, Nutrition, and the Thyroid: The Why, the Wherefore, and the Wiring." *Journal of Clinical Investigation* 105, no. 7 (April 2000): 859–61.

Forouzan, Iraj, and Mabel M. Bonilla. "Dystocia." *E-Medicine.* http://www.emedicine.com/med/topic3280.htm (accessed October 20, 2008).

Foster, Russell G., and Leon Kreitzman. *Rhythms of Life: The Biological Clocks That Control the Daily Lives of Every Living Thing.* New Haven, CT: Yale University Press, 2004.

Freedman, D. M., M. Dosemeci, and K. McGlynn. "Sunlight and Mortality from Breast, Ovarian, Colon, Prostate, and Non-melanoma Skin Cancer: A Composite Death Certificate Based Case-Control Study." *Occupational and Environmental Medicine* 59 (2002): 257–62.

Friedl, Erika. *Women of Deh Koh: Lives in an Iranian Village.* New York: Penguin, 1989.

Fulgoni, V., J. Nicholls, A. Reed, et al. "Dairy Consumption and Related Nutrient Intake in African-American Adults and Children in the United States: Continuing Survey of Food Intakes by Individuals 1994–1996, 1998, and the National Health and Nutrition Examination Survey 1999–2000." *Journal of the American Dietetics Association* 107, no. 2 (February 2007): 256–64.

Fuller, Kathleen E. "Health Disparities: Reframing the Problem." *Medical Science Monitor* 9, no. 3, special report (March 2003): SR9–15. Funk, Casimir. *Journal of State Medicine* 20 (1912): 341.

Garland, Cedric F. "More on Preventing Skin Cancer." *British Medical Journal* 327 (December 22, 2003): 1228.

Garland, Cedric F., and F. C. Garland. "Do Sunlight and Vitamin D Reduce the Likelihood of Colon Cancer?" *International Journal of Epidemiology* 9 (1980): 227–31.

Garland, Cedric F., Frank C. Garland, and Edward D. Gorham. "Calcium and Vitamin D: Their Potential Roles in Colon and Breast Cancer Prevention." *Annals of the New* York Academy of Sciences (1999): 107–19.

Garner, P., M. S. Kramer, and I. Chalmers. "Might Efforts to Increase Birthweight in

Undernourished Women Do More Harm Than Good?" *Lancet* 340, no. 8826 (October 24, 1999): 1021–23.

Garrison, Fielding. *An Introduction to the History of Medicine*. Philadelphia: W. B. Saunders Company, 1929.

Garzon, Philippe, and Mark J. Eisenberg. "Variation in the Mineral Content of Commercially Available Bottled Waters: Implications for Health and Disease." *American Journal of Medicine* 105 (August 1998): 125–30.

Gillie, Oliver. *Sunlight Robbery*. London: Health Research Forum, 2004.

"Global Dimming." BBC, *Science and Nature*, January 15, 2005. http://news.bbc.co.uk/2/hi/science/nature/4171591.stm (accessed October 21, 2008).

Gloth, F. M., III, W. Alam, and B. Hollis. "Vitamin D vs. Broad Spectrum Phototherapy in the Treatment of Seasonal Affective Disorder." *Journal of Nutritional Health and Aging* 3, no. 1 (1999): 5–7.

Gorham, E. D., F. C. Garland, and C. F. Garland. "Sunlight and Breast Cancer Incidence in the USSR." *International Journal of Epidemiology* 19 (1990): 820–24.

Goulding, A. "Children Who Avoid Drinking Cow's Milk Are at Increased Risk for Prepubertal Bone Fractures." *Journal of the American Dietetic Association* 104, no. 2 (2004): 250–53.

Grady, Denise. "After Caesareans, Some See Higher Insurance Cost." *New York Times.* http://www.nytimes.com/2008/06/01/health/01insure.html?_r=1 (accessed on October 13, 2008).

Grant, William. "An Ecologic Study of Dietary and Solar Ultraviolet-B Links to Breast Carcinoma Mortality Rates." *Cancer* 94, no. 1 (January 2002): 272–81.

Graves, Paul. "New Models and Metaphors for the Neanderthal Debate." *Current Anthropology* 32, no. 5 (December 1991): 513–41.

Greenlee, H., E. White, R. E. Patterson, et al. "Supplement Use among Cancer Survivors in the Vitamins and Lifestyle (VITAL) Study Cohort." *Journal of Alternative and Complementary Medicine* 10, no. 4 (August 2004): 660–66.

Grieser, Claudia M., Eberhard M. Greiser, and Martina Doren. "Menopausal Hormone Therapy and Risk of Ovarian Cancer: A Systematic Review." *Human Reproduction Update* 13, no. 5 (September/October 2007): 453–63.

Griffin, Dale W., Virginia H. Garrison, Jay R. Herman, and Eugene A. Shinn. "African Desert Dust in the Caribbean Atmosphere: Microbiology and Public Health." *Aerobiologia* 17 (2001): 203–13.

Griffin, Dale W., and Christina A. Kellogg. "Dust Storms and Their Impact on Ocean and Human Health: Dust in Earth's Atmosphere." *EcoHealth* 1 (July 13, 2004): 284–95.

Gross, Coleman, Donna M. Peehl, and David Feldman. "Vitamin D and Prostate Cancer." In *Vitamin D*, 2nd ed., edited by D. Feldman, F. H. Glorieux, and J. W. Pike. San Diego: Academic Press, 1997.

Guyton, Kathryn Z., Thomas W. Kensler, and Gary H. Posner. "Vitamin D and Vitamin

D Analogs as Cancer Chemopreventive Agents." *Nutrition Reviews* 61, no. 7 (July 2003): 227–37.

Halleran, Margaret M. "The Effect of Rickets on the Mental Development of Young Children." *Archives of Psychology* (July 1938): 5–61.

Hallfrisch, Judith G. "Boning Up on Navajo Food Habits." *Agricultural Research* (June 2001).

Hallfrisch, J., C. Veillon, K. Y. Patterson, A. D. Hill, I. Benn, B. Holiday, R. Burns, S. Zhonnie, F. Price, and A. Sorenson. "Bone-Related Mineral Content of Water Samples Collected on the Navajo Reservation." *Toxicology* 149, nos. 2–3 (August 21, 2000): 143–48.

Hamilton, Jon. "Pollution Found to Inhibit Rainfall in China." NPR, March 8, 2007. http://www.npr.org/templates/story/story.php?storyId=7779885 (accessed October 22, 2008).

Hamoui, N., G. Anthone, and P. F. Crooks. "Calcium Metabolism in the Morbidly Obese." *Obesity Surgery* 14, no. 1 (January 2004): 9–12.

Haney, E., M. Haney, D. Stadler, and M. M. Bliziotes. "Vitamin D Insufficiency in Internal Medicine Residents." *Calcified Tissue International* 76, no. 1 (January 2005): 11–16.

Harris, Diane M., and Vay Liang W. Go. "Vitamin D and Colon Carcinogenesis." *Journal of Nutrition* 134, suppl. (December 2004): 3463S–71S.

Harris, Leslie J. *Vitamins: A Digest of Current Knowledge.* London: J. & A. Churchill, Ltd., 1951.

Hatun, Sukru, Behzat Ozkan, Zerrin Orbak, et al. "Vitamin D Deficiency in Early Infancy." *Journal of Nutrition* 135 (February 2005): 279–82.

Hayes, C. E. "Vitamin D: A Natural Inhibitor of Multiple Sclerosis." *Proceedings of Nutrition Society* 59, no. 4 (2000): 531–35.

Heaney, Robert P. "Functional Indices of Vitamin D Status and Ramifications of Vitamin D Deficiency." *American Journal of Clinical Nutrition* 80, suppl. (2004): 1706S–1709S.

Heininger, Kurt. "A Unifying Hypothesis of Alzheimer's Disease; Risk Factors." *Human Psychopharmacology: Clinical and Experimental* 15, no. 1 (March 7, 2000): 1–70.

Henderson, R. J., C. M. Frampton, M. D. Thomas, and C. T. Eason. "Field Evaluations of Cholecalciferol, Gliftor, and Brodifacoum for the Control of Brushtail Possums (*Trichosurus vulpecula*). *New Zealand Journal of Agricultural Research* 39, no. 3 (September 1996): 397–400.

Henriksen, T., A. Dahlback, S. H. Larsen, and J. Moan. "Ultraviolet-Radiation and Skin Cancer. Effect of an Ozone Layer Depletion." *Photochemistry and Photobiology* 51, no. 5 (May 1990): 579–82.

Henschen, Folke. *The History and Geography of Diseases.* Translated by Joan Tate. New York: Delacorte Press, 1966.

Herodotus. *The Histories*. Translated by Robin Waterfield. New York: Oxford University Press, 1998.

Hershberger, P. A., R. A. Modzelewski, Z. R. Shurin, et al. "1,25-Dihydroxycholecalciferol (1,25-D3) Inhibits the Growth of Squamous Cell Carcinoma and Down-Modulates p21Waf1/Cip1 in Vitro and in Vivo." *Cancer Research* 59, no. 11 (June 1, 1999): 2644–49.

Hess, A. F. "Infantile Scurvy: Its Influence on Growth." *American Journal of Diseases of Children* (August 1916): 152–65.

Hess, A. F., and M. Fish. "Scurvy in Children." *American Journal of Disabled Children* 8 (1914): 386.

Hicks, G. J., J. W. Davis, and R. A. Hicks. "Fatal Alcohol-Related Traffic Crashes Increase Subsequent to Changes to and from Daylight Savings Time." *Perceptual Motor Skills* 86, no. 3 pt. 1 (June 1998): 879–82.

Hillman, Mayer, and Jon Parker. "Communications: More Daylight, Less Electricity." *Energy Policy* 16, no. 5 (October 1988): 514–15.

"History of Flaksted and Moskenes, Lofoten Islands, Norway." http://www.lofoten-info.no/history.htm#5 (accessed October 21, 2008).

Hobday, Richard. *The Healing Sun: Sunlight and Health in the Twenty-first Century*. London: Findhorn Press, 2000.

Hochwald, O., I. Harman-Boehm, and H. Castel. "Hypovitaminosis D among Inpatients in a Sunny Country." *Israel Medical Association Journal* 6, no. 2 (February 2004): 82–87.

Hockberger, Philip E. "A History of Ultraviolet Photobiology for Humans, Animals and Microorganisms." *Photochemistry and Photobiology* 76, no. 6 (December 2002): 561–79.

Holick, Michael F. "Calcium and Vitamin D, Diagnostics and Therapeutics." *Clinical Laboratory Medicine* 20, no. 3 (September 2000): 569–90.

———. "Vitamin D: A Millenium Perspective." *Journal of Cellular Biochemistry* 88, no. 2: 296–307

Holick, Michael F., and Mark Jenkins. *The UV Advantage*. New York: Ibooks, 2003.

Horst, Ronald L., and Timothy A. Reinhardt. "Vitamin D Metabolism." In *Vitamin D*, 2nd ed., edited by D. Feldman, F. H. Glorieux, and J. W. Pike. San Diego: Academic Press, 1997.

Hu, Frank B., Meir J. Stampfer, JoAnn E. Manson, et al. "Dietary Fat Intake and the Risk of Coronary Heart Disease in Women." *New England Journal of Medicine* 337, no. 21 (November 20, 1997): 1491–99.

Hughes, A. M., B. K. Armstrong, C. M. Vajdic, et al. "Sun Exposure May Protect against Non-Hodgkin Lymphoma: A Case-Control Study." *International Journal of Cancer* 112, no. 5 (December 10, 2004): 865–71.

Huldschinsky, Kurt. "Preventive Irradiation of Children against Rickets." *British Journal of Actinotherapy* (September 1928): 103–105.

Hutt, M. S. R., and D. P. Burkitt. *The Geography of Non-Infectious Disease.* New York: Oxford University Press, 1986.

Hypponen, E. "Micronutrients and the Risk of Type 1 Diabetes: Vitamin D, Vitamin E, and Nicotinamide." *Nutrition Review* 62, no. 9 (September 2004): 340–47.

Hypponen, E., E. Laara, A. Reunanen, M. R. Jarvelin, and S. M. Virtanen. "Intake of Vitamin D and Risk of Type 1 Diabetes; A Birth-Cohort Study." *Lancet* 358, no. 9292 (November 3, 2001): 1500–1503.

Imataka, G., T. Mikami, H. Yamanouchi, K. Kano, and M. Eguchi. "Vitamin D Deficiency Rickets Due to Soybean Milk." *Journal of Pediatric Child Health* (March 3, 2004): 154–55.

International Relations and Security Network, Center for Security Studies, Zurich, Switzerland. http://www.isn.ethz.ch/researchpub/publihouse/za_cbw/ (accessed October 21, 2008).

Jolly, S. E., C. T. Eason, and C. Frampton. "Serum Calcium Levels in Response to Cholecalciferol and Calcium Carbonate in the Australian Brushtail Possum." *Pesticide Biochemistry Physiology* 47 (1993): 159–64.

Kamycheva, Elena, Ragnar M. Joakimsen, and Rolf Jorde. "Intakes of Calcium and Vitamin D Predict Body Mass Index in the Population of Northern Norway." *Journal of Nutrition* 133 (January 2003): 102–106.

Kannus, P., K. Uusi-Rasi, M. Palvanen, and J. Parkkari. "Non-Pharmacological Means to Prevent Fractures among Older Adults." *Annals of Medicine* 37, no. 4 (2005): 303–10.

Kawasaki, I. "Intake of Vitamin D and Muscular Volume." *Clinical Calcium* 15, no. 9 (September 2005): 1517–21.

Keane, E. M., M. Healy, R. O'Moore, D. Coakley, and J. B. Walsh. "Vitamin-D Fortified Liquid Milk: Benefits for the Elderly Community-Based Population." *Calcified Tissue International* 62 (1998): 300–302.

Khawaja, M., R. Jurdi, and T. Kabakian-Khasholian. "Rising Trends in Cesarean Section Rates in Egypt." *Birth* 31, no. 1 (March 31, 2004): 12–16.

Ko, P., R. Burkert, J. McGrath, and D. Eyles. "Maternal Vitamin D(3) Deprivation and the Regulation of Apoptosis and Cell Cycle during Rat Brain Development." *Developmental Brain Research* 153, no. 1 (October 15, 2004): 61–68.

Kobayashi, Masako, and Maiko Kobayashi. "The Relationship between Obesity and Seasonal Variation in Body Weight among Elementary School Children in Tokyo." *Economics and Human Biology* 4, no. 2 (June 2006): 253–61.

Kohnen, L., and J. Magotteaux. "Acute and Recurrent Night Leg Pain in Young Children: 'Growing Pains.'" *Revue Medical de Liege* 59, no. 6 (June 2004): 363–66.

Konje, Justin C., and Oladapo A. Ladipo. "Nutrition and Obstructed Labor." *American Journal of Clinical Nutrition* 72, suppl. (2000): 291S–97S.

Koutkia, P., Z. Lu, T. C. Chen, and M. F. Holick. "Treatment of Vitamin D Deficiency Due to Crohn's Disease with Tanning Bed Ultraviolet B Radiation." *Gastroenterology* 121, no. 6 (December 2001): 1485–88.

Krause, R., M. Buhring, W. Hopfenmuller, M. F. Holick, and A. M. Sharma. "Ultraviolet B and Blood Pressure." *Lancet* 352, no. 9129 (1998): 709–10.

Kraut, Alan. "Dr. Joseph Goldberger and the War on Pellagra." National Institutes of Health. http://history.nih.gov/exhibits/Goldberger/full-text.htm (accessed October 21, 2008).

Kreider, Jan F. and Frank Kreith, ed. *Solar Energy Handbook*. New York: McGraw-Hill, 1981.

Kumar, Rajiv, ed. *Vitamin D: Basic and Clinical Aspects*. Boston: Martinus Nijhoff Publishing, 1984.

Kunz, D. "Chronobiotic Protocol and Circadian Sleep Propensity Index: New Tools for Clinical Routine and Research on Melatonin and Sleep." *Pharmacopsychiatry* 37 no. 4 (July 2004): 139–46.

Kurlansky, Mark. *Cod: A Biography of the Fish That Changed the World*. New York: Penguin, 1997.

Kutluk, G., F. Cetinkaya, and M. Basak. "Comparisons of Oral Calcium, High Dose Vitamin D and a Combination of These in the Treatment of Nutritional Rickets in Children." *Journal of Tropical Pediatrics* 48, no. 6 (2002): 351–53.

Laing, Gordon J. *Survivals of Roman Religion.* New York: Longmans, 1931.

Landsdowne, A. T., and S. C. Provost. "Vitamin D3 Enhances Mood in Healthy Subjects during Winter." *Psychopharmacology* 135, no. 4 (February 1998): 319–23.

Lane, N. E., L. R. Gore, S. R. Cummings, et al. "Serum Vitamin D Levels and Incident Changes of Radiographic Hip Osteoarthritis: A Longitudinal Study." Study of Osteoporotic Fractures Research Group. *Arthritis and Rheumatism* 42, no. 5 (1999): 854–60.

Large, D. M., E. B. Mawer, and M. Davies. "Dystrophic Calcification, Cataracts, and Enamel Hypoplasia Due to Long-Standing, Privational Vitamin D Deficiency." *Metabolic Bone Disease Related Research* 5, no. 5 (1984): 215–18.

Larkin, Marilynn, "How Green Is Your Workout?" *Lancet* 355 (2000): 1702–1703.

Lau, E. M. C., H. Lynn, and J. Woo. "Milk Supplementation Prevents Loss in Postmenopausal Chinese Women Over 3 Years." *Bone* 32 (2002): 536–40.

Lazovich, DeAnn, et al. "Characteristics Associated with Use or Intention to Use Indoor Tanning among Adolescents." *Archives of Pediatrics and Adolescent Medicine* 158, no. 9 (September 2004).

Leas, Connie. *Fat: It's Not What You Think*. Amherst, NY: Prometheus Books, 2008.

Lefkowitz, E. S., and C. F. Garland. "Sunlight, Vitamin D, and Ovarian Cancer Mortality Rates in U.S. Women." *International Journal of Epidemiology* 23 (1994): 1133–36.

Lehrer, Michael S., and Alain Rook. "Extracorporeal Photopheresis." December 3, 2004. www.emedicine.com/derm/topic566.htm (accessed October 21, 2008).

Levine, Victor E. "Sunlight and Its Many Values." *Scientific Monthly* 29, no. 6 (December 1929).

Lewis, Simon L., Yadvinder Malhi, and Oliver L. Phillips. "Fingerprinting the Impacts of Global Change on Tropical Forests." *Philosophical Transactions: Biological Sciences* 359, no. 1443 (March 29, 2004): 437–62.

Lewis, Simon L., O. L. Phillips, T. R. Baker, et al. "Concerted Changes in Tropical Forest Structure and Dynamids: Evidence from 50 South American Long-Term Plots." *Philosophical Transactions: Biological Sciences* 359, no. 1443 (March 2004): 421–36.

Lewy, A. J., T. A. Wehr, F. K. Goodwin, D. A. Newsome, and S. P, Markey. "Light Suppresses Melatonin Secretion in Humans." *Science* 210, no. 4475 (December 12, 1980): 1267–69.

Liberman, Jacob. *Light: Medicine of the Future.* Rochester, VT: Bear and Company, 1991.

Liepert, Beate G. "Observed Reductions of Surface Solar Radiation at Sites in the United States and Worldwide from 1961 to 1990." *Geophysical Research Letters* (April 2002).

Lillyquist, Michael J. *Sunlight and Health: The Positive and Negative Effects of the Sun on You.* New York: Dodd, Mead, and Company, 1985.

Lim, H. W., and R. L. Edelson. "Photopheresis for the Treatment of Cutaneous T-Cell Lymphoma." *Hematology Oncology Clinician North America* 9, no. 5 (October 1995): 117–26.

Lin, R., and J. H. White. "The Pleiotropic Actions of Vitamin D." *Bioessays* 26, no. 1 (January 2004): 21–28.

Littleton, C. Scott. *Mythology: The Illustrated Anthology of World Myth & Storytelling.* London: Duncan Baird Publishers, 2002.

Lorber, Jakob. *The Healing Power of Sunlight.* Salt Lake City: Merkur Publishing, 2000.

Lutila, Terhi A., et al. "Bioavailability of Vitamin D from Wild Edible Mushrooms (*Cantharellus tubaeformis*) as Measured with a Human Bioassay." *American Journal of Clinical Nutrition* 69 (1999): 95–98.

Macchi, M. M., and J. N. Bruce. "Human Pineal Physiology and Functional Significance of Melatonin." *Frontiers in Neuroendocrinology* 25, nos. 3–4 (September/December 2004): 177–95.

MacDill, Marjorie. "Babies in Old Paintings Had Rickets." *Science News-Letter* (March 17, 1928): 163–66.

————. "Dinosaurs Died of Rickets." *Science News-Letter* (August 4, 1928): 63–64.

Mackay-Sim, A., F. Feron, D. Eyles, T. Burne, and J. McGrath. "Schizophrenia, Vitamin D, and Brain Development." *International Review of Neurobiology* 59 (2004): 351–80.

Mahoney, Sheila F., and Lorraine Halinka Malcoe. "Cesarean Delivery in Native American Women: Are Low Rates Explained by Practices Common to the Indian Health Service?" *Birth* 32, no. 3 (September 2005): 170–78.

Manners, P. "Are Growing Pains a Myth?" *Australian Family Physician* 28, no. 2 (February 1999): 124–27.

Marshall, Trevor G. "Vitamin D Discovery Outpaces FDA Decision Making." *BioEssays* 30, no. 2 (January 15, 2008): 173–82.

Martin, R., P. P. Foels, G. Clanton, and K. Moon. "Season of Birth Is Related to Child Retention Rates, Achievement, and Rate of Diagnosis of Specific LD." *Journal of Learning Disabilities* 37, no. 4 (July/August 2004): 307–17.

Marwick, Charles. "New Light on Skin Cancer Mechanisms." *Journal of the American Medical Association* 274, no. 6 (August 9, 1995): 445–46.

Mascarenahas, R., and S. Mobarhan. "Hypovitaminosis D-Induced Pain." *Nutrition Reviews* 62, no. 9 (September 2004): 354–59.

Mason, R. S. "Vitamin D: New Insights into an Old Secosteroid." *Asia Pacific Journal of Clinical Nutrition* 14, suppl. (2005): S19.

Mather, Cotton. *Angel of Bethesda.* Edited by Gordon W. Jones. Barre, MA: American Antiquarian Society, 1972.

Matkovic, V., J. Z. Ilich, N. E. Badenhop, M. Skugor, A. Clairmont, D. Klisovic, and J. D. Landoll. "Gain in Body Fat Is Inversely Related to the Nocturnal Rise in Serum Leptin Level in Young Females." *Journal of Clinical Endocrinology and Metabolism* 82, no. 5 (1997): 1368–72.

Mattila, C., P. Knekt, S. Mannisto, et al. "Serum 25-Hydroxyvitamin D Concentration and Subsequent Risk of Type 2 Diabetes." *Diabetes Care* 30 (2007): 2569–70.

Mayer, Jean, and Johanna T. Dwyer, eds. *Food and Nutrition Policy in a Changing World.* New York: Oxford University Press, 1979.

Mayron, L.W., J. N. Ott, E. J. Amontree, and R. Nations. "Caries Reduction in School Children." *Applied Radiology* (July/August 1975): 56–58.

————. "Light, Radiation, and Dental Caries." *Academic Therapy* 10 (1975): 441–48.

McAlindon, T. E., D. T. Felson, Y. Zhang, et al. "Relation of Dietary Intake and Serum Levels of Vitamin D to Progression of Osteoarthritis of the Knee among Participants in the Framingham Study." *Annals of Internal Medicine* 125, no. 5 (1996): 353–59.

McBeath, E. C., and T. F. Zucker. "The Role of Vitamin D in the Control of Dental Caries in Children." *Journal of Nutrition* 15, no. 6 (1938): 547–64.

McCarty, M. F., and C. A. Thomas. "PTH Excess May Promote Weight Gain by

Impeding Catecholamine-Induced Lipolysis: Implications for the Impact of Calcium, Vitamin D, and Alcohol on Body Weight." *Medical Hypotheses* 61, nos. 5–6 (November/December 2003): 535–42.

McCollum, Elmer Verner. *A History of Nutrition*. Boston: Houghton Mifflin, 1957.

McCollum, E. V., and M. Davis. "The Necessity of Certain Lipids in the Diet during Growth." *Journal of Biological Chemistry* 15 (1915): 167–75.

McCollum, E. V., N. Simmonds, J. E. Becker, and P. G. Shipley. "Studies on Experimental Rickets." *Journal of Biological Chemistry* 53 (1922): 293–312.

McEnany, Geoffry, and Kathryn A. Lee. "Owls, Larks and the Significance of Morningness/Eveningness Rhythm Propensity in Psychiatric-Mental Health Nursing." *Issues in Mental Health Nursing* 21, no. 2 (March 1, 2000): 203–16.

McGrath, J. "Does 'Imprinting' with Low Prenatal Vitamin D Contribute to the Risk of Various Adult Disorders?" *Medical Hypotheses* 56 no. 3 (Mar. 2001): 367–71.

McGrath, John, Darryl Eyles, B. Mowry, R. Yolken, and S. Buka. "Low Maternal Vitamin D as a Risk Factor for Schizophrenia; A Pilot Study Using Banked Sera." *Schizophrenia Research* 63, nos. 1–2 (September 1, 2003): 73–78.

McGrath, John, K. Saari, H. Hakko, J. Jokelainen, P. Jones, M. R. Jarvelin, D. Chant, and M. Isohanni. "Vitamin D Supplementation during the First Year of Life and Risk of Schizophrenia: A Finnish Birth Cohort Study." *Schizophrenia Research* 67, nos. 2–3 (April 1, 2004): 237–45.

McGrath, J. J., S. Saha, D. E. Lieberman, and S. Buka. "Season of Birth Is Associated with Anthropometric and Neurocognitive Outcomes during Infancy and Childhood in a General Population Birth Cohort." *Schizophrenia Research* 81, no. 1 (January 2006): 91–100.

McGregor, Deborah Kuhn. *From Midwives to Medicine: The Birth of American Gynecology*. New Brunswick, NJ: Rutgers University Press, 1998.

McKenna, M. J., R. Freaney, P. Byrne, et al. "Safety and Efficacy of Increasing Wintertime Vitamin D and Calcium Intake by Milk Fortification." *Quarterly Journal of Medicine* 88 (1995): 895–98.

Meade, Melinda, John Florin, and Wilbert Gesler. *Medical Geography*. New York: Guilford Press, 1988.

Melamed, M. L., E. D. Michos, W. Post, and B. Astor. "25-Hydroxyvitamin D Levels and the Risk of Mortality in the General Population." *Archives of Internal Medicine* 168, no. 15 (August 11, 2008): 1629–37.

Mellanby, Edward. *A Story of Nutritional Research: The Effect of Some Dietary Factors on Bones and the Nervous System*. Baltimore: Williams and Wilkins Co., 1950.

———. "Progress in Medical Science." In *Scientific Progress*. Edited by James Jeans et al. New York: Macmillan, 1936.

Mellanby, May. "An Experimental Study of the Influence of Diet on Teeth Formation." *Lancet* (December 7, 1918): 767–70.

Micronutrient Information Center. Linus Pauling Institute. Oregon State University, Corvallis. http://lpi.oregonstate.edu/infocenter/vitamins/vitaminD/ (accessed October 21, 2008).

Miller, C. G., and W. Chutkan. "Vitamin-D Deficiency Rickets in Jamaican Children." *Archives of Disease in Childhood* 51, no. 3 (March 1976): 214–18.

"Million Reported Bid for Vitamin D Rights." *New York Times*, February 13, 1931, 21:4.

Mitchell, R. A. C., C. L. Gibbard, F. J. Mitchell, and D. W. Lawlor. "Effects of Shading in Different Developmental Phases on Biomass and Grain Yield of Winter Wheat at Ambient and Elevated CO2." *Plant Cell and Environment.* http://www.blackwell publishing.com/journal.asp?ref=0140-7791&site=1 (accessed October 21, 2008).

Moon, S. J., A. A. Fryer, and R. C. Strange. "Ultraviolet Radiation, Vitamin D and Prostate Cancer Risk." *Photochemistry and Photobiology* (January 1, 2005).

Morrow, Carla. "Cholecalciferol Poisoning." *Veterinary Medicine* (December 2001).

Mtimavalye, L. A., C. D. van der Does, and J. B. Maathuis. "The Relationship between Increasing Birthweight and Cephalopelvic Disproportion in Dar es Salaam, Tanzania." *Journal of Obstetrics and Gynaecology of the British Commonwealth* 81, no. 5 (May 1974): 380–82.

Munger, K. L., S. M. Zhang, E. O'Reilly, et al. "Vitamin D Intake and Incidence of Multiple Sclerosis." *Neurology* 62 (January 13, 2004): 60–65.

Natri, Anna-Mari, et al. "Bread Fortified with Cholecalciferol Increases the Serum 25-Hydroxyvitamin D Concentration in Women as Effectively as a Cholecalciferol Supplement." *Journal of Nutrition* 136 (2006): 123–27.

Need, A. G., H. A. Morris, M. Horowitz, and C. Nordin. "Effects of Skin Thickness, Age, Body Fat, and Sunlight on Serum 25-Hydroxyvitamin D." *American Journal of Clinical Nutrition* 58, no. 6 (December 1993): 882–85.

Neilson, J. P., T. Lavender, S. Quenby, and S. Wray. "Obstructed Labour." *British Medical Bulletin* 67 (2003): 191–204.

Newmark, Martin S., Harold L. Newmark, Gary Kelloff, and Martin Lipkin. *Calcium, Vitamin D, and Prevention of Colon Cancer*. Boca Raton, FL: CRC Press, 1991.

Nobel Foundation. *Physiology or Medicine*. Vol. 1. New York: Elsevier, 1967.

Normal, P. E., and J. T. Powell. "Vitamin D, Shedding Light on the Development of Disease in Peripheral Arteries." *Arteriosclerosis, Thrombosis, and Vascular Biology* 25 (2005): 39.

Norman, Anthony W., ed. *Vitamin D: Molecular Biology and Clinical Nutrition* New York: Marcel Dekker, 1980.

———. *Vitamin D: The Calcium Homeostatic Steroid Hormone*. New York: Academic Press, 1979.

Oberklaid, F., D. Amos, C. Liu, F. Jarman, A. Sanson, and M. Prior. "Growing Pains: Clinical and Behavioral Correlates in a Community Sample." *Journal of Developmental and Behavioral Pediatrics* 18, no. 2 (April 1997): 102–106.

Oboh, Alex, and Babatunde A. Gbolade. "Correspondence." *BJOG: International Journal of Obstetrics and Gynaecology* 110, no. 8 (August 2003): 787–88.

O'Hara, Gwydion. *Sun Lore: Folktales and Sagas from around the World.* St. Paul: Llewellyn Publications, 1997.

Olcott, William Tyler. *Sun Lore of All Ages.* New York: G. P. Putnam's Sons, 1914.

Olders, H. "Average Sunrise Time Predicts Depression Prevalence." *Journal of Psychosomatic Research* 55, no. 2 (August 2003): 99–105.

Osborne, Michael, Peter Boyle, and Martin Lipkin. "Cancer Prevention." *Lancet* 349, suppl. 2 (1997): 27–30.

Ott, John N. *Health and Light: The Effects of Natural and Artificial Light on Man and Other Living Things.* Greenwich, CN: Devin-Adair Co., 1973.

Ovesen, L., R. Andersen, and J. Jakobsen. "Geographical Differences in Vitamin D Status, with Particular Reference to European Countries." *Proceedings of the Nutrition Society* 62, no. 4 (November 2003): 813–21.

Oyakhire, G. K. "Environmental Factors Influencing Maternal Mortality in Zaria, Nigeria." *Rural Sociology Health Journal* 100, no. 2 (April 1980): 72–74.

Palm, Theobald A. "The Geographical Distribution and Etiology of Rickets." *Practitioner* 45 (October 1890): 270–79; (November 1890): 321–42.

Palmer, Douglas. "Big Chill Killed Off the Neanderthals." *New Scientist* (January 24 2004): 10–11.

Palmer, N. B., and J. D. Palmer. "The Dental Caries Experience of 5-, 12- and 14-Year-Old Children in Great Britain." Surveys coordinated by the British Association for the Study of Community Dentistry in 1990–91, 1991–92, and 1992–93. *Community Dental Health* 11, no. 1 (1994): 42–52.

Park, S., and M. A. Johnson. "Living in Low-Latitude Regions in the United States Does Not Prevent Poor Vitamin D Status." *Nutrition Reviews* 63, no. 6 pt. 1 (June 2005): 203–209.

Peplonska, B., J. Lissowska, T. J. Hartman, et al. "Adulthood Lifetime Physical Activity and Breast Cancer," *Epidemiology* 19, no. 2 (March 2008): 226–36.

Peterson, H. A. "Leg Aches." *Pediatric Clinics of North America* 24, no. 4 (November 1977): 731–36.

Peterson, Norma. "The Sunshine Factor: Vitamin D and Breast Cancer." *Breast Cancer Action Network Newsletter* 12 (June 2002): 12.

Pettifor, J. M., P. Ross, and J. Wang. "Rickets in Children of Rural Origin in South Africa: Is Dietary Calcium a Factor?" *Journal of Pediatrics* 92, no. 2 (1978): 320–24.

Pfeifer, M., B. Begerow, H. W. Minne, D. Nachtigall, and C. Hansen. "Effects of a Short-Term Vitamin D3 and Calcium Supplementation on Blood Pressure and Parathyroid Hormone Levels in Elderly Women." *Journal Clinical Endocrinology Metabolism* 86, no. 4 (2001): 1633–37.

Ping-Delfos, W. C., et al. "Acute Suppression of Spontaneous Food Intake Following Dairy Calcium and Vitamin D." *Asian Pacific Journal of Clinical Nutrition* 13, suppl. (2004): S82.

Plotnikoff, Gregory A., and Joanna M. Quigley. "Prevalence of Severe Hypovitaminosis D in Patients with Persistent, Nonspecific Musculoskeletal Pain." *Mayo Clinic Proceedings* 78, no. 12 (December 2003): 1463.

Ponsonby, Anne-Louise, Anthony McMichael, and Ingrid van der Mei. "Ultraviolet Radiation and Autoimmune Disease: Insights from Epidemiological Research." *Toxicology* 181–82 (2002): 71–78.

Porter, Roy. *The Greatest Benefit to Mankind.* New York: Norton, 1997.

"Portrait of a Neanderthal." *New Scientist* (July 24, 2004): 17.

Potter, J. E., E. Berquo, I. H. Perpetuo, O. F. Leal, K. Hopkins, M. R. Souza, and M. C. Formiga. "Unwanted Caesarean Sections among Public and Private Patients in Brazil: Prospective Study." *British Medical Journal* 323, no. 7322 (November 17, 2001): 1155–58.

Price, Weston A. *Nutrition and Physical Degeneration.* La Mesa, CA: Price-Pottenger Nutrition Foundation, 2003.

Pringsheim, Tamara. "Cluster Headache: Evidence for a Disorder of Circadian Rhythm and Hypothalamic Function." *Canadian Journal of Neurological Sciences* 29 (2002): 33–40.

"Produce New Bread with Vitamin D." *New York Times*, February 12, 1931, 2:5.

Pruitt, Ida. *A Daughter of Han: The Autobiography of a Chinese Working Woman.* Stanford, CA: Stanford University Press, 1967.

Przybelski, P. R., S. Agrawal, D. Krueger, J. A. Engelke, F. Walbrun, and N. Binkley. "Rapid Correction of Low Vitamin D Status in Nursing Home Residents." *Osteoporosis International* (April 2008).

Pugliese, M. T., D. L. Blumberg, J. Hudzinski, and S. Kay. "Nutritional Rickets in Suburbia." *Journal of American College of Nutrition* 17, no. 6 (December 1998): 637–41.

Raiten, Daniel J., and Mary Frances Picciano. "Vitamin D and Health in the 21st Century: Bone and Beyond." Executive summary. *American Journal of Clinical Nutrition* 80, suppl. (2004): 1673S–77S.

Rajakumar, K., and S. B. Thomas. "Reemerging Nutritional Rickets: A Historical Perspective." *Archives of Pediatric Adolescent Medicine* 159, no. 4 (April 2005): 335–41.

"Rates of Cesarean Delivery: United States, 1991." Office of Vital and Health Statistics Systems, National Center for Health Statistics, Centers for Disease Control. http://www.cdc.gov/mmwr/preview/mmwrhtml/00020285.htm (accessed October 21, 2008).

Reiter, R. J., et al. "Light at Night, Chronodisruption, Melatonin Suppression, and Cancer

Risk: A Review." *Critical Reviews in Oncogenesis* 13, no. 4 (2007): 303–28.

Rejnmark, L., M. E. Jorgensen, M. B. Pedersen, et al. "Vitamin D Insufficiency in Greenlanders on a Westernized Fare; Ethnic Differences in Calcitropic Hormones between Greenlanders and Danes." *Calcified Tissue International* 74, no. 3 (March 2004): 255–63.

Rhodes, Lesley E., Brian H. Durham, William D. Fraser, and Peter S. Friedmann. "Dietary Fish Oil Reduces Basal and Ultraviolet B-Generated PGE$_2$ Levels in Skin and Increases the Threshold to Provocation of Polymorphic Light Eruption." *Journal of Investigative Dermatology* 105, no. 4 (October 1995): 532–35.

Roberts, John S., et al. "Vitamin D$_2$ Formation from Post-harvest UV-B Treatment of Mushrooms (*Agaricus bisporus*) and Retention during Storage." *Journal of Agricultural Food Chemistry* 56, no. 12 (2008): 4541–44.

Roderick, M. L., and G. D. Farquahar. "Changes in Australian Pan Evaporation from 1970 to 2002." *International Journal of Climatology* 24, no. 9 (July 2004): 1077–90.

Roe, Daphne. *A Plague of Corn; The Social History of Pellagra.* Ithaca, NY: Cornell University Press, 1973.

Romano, T. J. "Fibromyalgia in Children; Diagnosis and Treatment." *West Virginia Medical Review* 87, no. 3 (March 1991): 112–14.

Rosenthal, Norman E. *Winter Blues: Seasonal Affective Disorder, What It Is and How to Overcome It.* New York: Guilford Press, 1998.

Rostand, S. G. "Ultraviolet Light May Contribute to Geographic and Racial Blood Pressure Differences." *Hypertension* 30, no. 2 pt. 1 (1997): 150–56.

Roux, S., C. Baudoin, D. Boute, M. Brazier, V. De La Gueronniere, M. C. De Vernejoul. "Biological Effects of Drinking-Water Mineral Composition on Calcium Balance and Bone Remodeling Markers." *Journal of Nutrition, Health & Aging* 8, no. 5 (2004): 380–84.

Rowe, Paul M. "Why Is Rickets Resurgent in the USA?" *Lancet* (April 7, 2001): 357.

Rucker, D., J. A. Allan, G. H. Fick, and D. A. Hanley. "Vitamin D Insufficiency in a Population of Healthy Western Canadians." *Canadian Medical Association Journal* 166, no. 12 (2002): 1517–24.

Saag, Kenneth G., et al. "Vitamin D Intake Is Inversely Associated with Rheumatoid Arthritis: Results from the Iowa Women's Health Study." *Arthritis and Rheumatism* 50 (January 2004): 72–77.

Sachan, Alok, Renu Gupta, Vinita Das, Anjoo Agarwal, Pradeep K. Awasthi, and Vijayalakshmi Bahtia. "High Prevalence of Vitamin D Deficiency among Pregnant Women and Their Newborns in Northern India." *American Journal of Clinical Nutrition* 81, no. 5 (May 2005): 1060–64.

Salamolun, M. M., A. S. Kizirian, R. I. Tannous, M. M. Nabulsi, M. K. Choucair, M. E. Deeb, and G. A. El-Haff Fuleihan. "Low Calcium and Vitamin D Intake in Healthy

Children and Adolescents and Their Correlates." *European Journal of Clinical Nutrition* (October 6, 2004).

Sandanger, T. M., M. Brustad, E. Lund, and I. C. Burkow. "Change in Levels of Persistent Organic Pollutants in Human Plasma after Consumption of a Traditional Northern Norwegian Fish Dish—Molje (Cod, Cod Liver, Cod Liver Oil and Hard Roe)." *Journal of Environmental Monitoring* 5, no. 1 (February 2003): 160–65.

Sasson, A., Z. Etzioni, S. Shany, G. M. Berlyne, and R. Yagil. "Growth and Bone Mineralisation as Affected by Dietary Calcium, Phytic Acid and Vitamin D." *Comparative Biochemistry and Physiology* 72, no. 1 (1982): 43–48.

Scanlon, Kelly S., ed. *Final Report.* Vitamin D Expert Panel Meeting, Atlanta, October 11–12, 2001.

Schooneman, F. "Extracorporeal Photopheresis Technical Aspects." *Transfusion Apheresis Science* 28, no. 1 (February 2003): 51–61.

Schrager, Sarina. "Dietary Calcium Intake and Obesity." *Journal of American Board of Family Practice* 18 (2005): 205–10.

Schulte, C. M. "Review Article: Bone Disease in Inflammatory Bowel Disease." *Alimentary Pharmacology Therapy* 20, suppl. (October 2004): 43–49.

Schwartz, G. G. "Vitamin D and the Epidemiology of Prostate Cancer." *Seminars in Dialysis* 18, no. 4 (July/August 2005): 276–89.

Schwartz, Joan. "Research Briefs." *Boston University Bridge*, May 15, 2003.

Sedrani, S. H. "Low 25-Hydroxyvitamin D and Normal Serum Calcium Concentrations in Saudi Arabia: Riyadh Region." *Annals of Nutrition and Metabolism* 28, no. 3 (1984): 181–85.

———. "Vitamin D Status of Saudi Men." *Tropical and Geographical Medicine* 36, no. 2 (June 1984): 181–87.

Sedrani, S. H., A. W. Alidrissy, and K. M. El Arabi. "Sunlight and Vitamin D Status in Normal Saudi Subjects." *American Journal of Clinical Nutrition* 38, no. 1 (July 1983): 129–32.

Seely, Stephen, David L. J. Freed, Gerald A. Silverstone, and Vicky Rippere. *Diet-Related Diseases: The Modern Epidemic.* Westport, CT: Avi, 1985.

"Sees Child Health Rising." *New York Times*, March 1, 1932, 10:7.

Sellers, Elizabeth A. C., Atul Sharma, and Celia Rodd. "Adaptation of Inuit Children to a Low-Calcium Diet." *Canadian Medical Association Journal* 168, no. 9 (April 29, 2003): 1141–43.

Semba, Richard D. "Vitamin A as 'Anti-Infective' Therapy, 1920–1940." *Journal of Nutrition* 129 (1999): 783–91.

Seres, A., A. Papp, and I. Suveges. "Photodynamic Therapy in Age-Related Macular Degeneration." *Orvosi Hetililap* 146, no. 42 (October 2005): 2143–49.

"Severe Malnutrition among Young Children; Georgia, January 1977–June 1999." *MMWR Weekly* 50, no. 12 (March 30, 2001): 224–27.

Shaw, N. J., and B. R. Pal. "Vitamin D Deficiency in UK Asian Families: Activating a New Concern." *Archives of Disease in Childhood* 86 (2002): 147–49.

Shiono, P. H., D. McNellis, and G. G. Rhoads. "Reasons for the Rising Cesarean Delivery Rates: 1978–1984." *Obstetrics and Gynecology* 69, no. 5 (May 1987): 696–700.

Shirima, C. P., and J. L. Kinabo. "Nutritional Status and Birth Outcomes of Adolescent Pregnant Girls in Morogoro, Coast, and Dar es Salaam Regions, Tanzania." *Nutrition* 21, no. 1 (January 2005): 32–38.

"Short-Wave Vitamins." *New York Times*, February 4, 1931, 24:4.

Sims, J. Marion. "Further Observations on Trismus Nascentium with Cases Illustrating Its Etiology and Treatment." *American Journal of the Medical Sciences* 16 (July 1848): 59–79.

———. *The Story of My Life*. Edited by J. Marion Sims. New York: D. Appleton, 1886.

Singh, Madanjeet. *The Sun: Symbol of Power and Life*. New York: Harry N. Abrams, 1993.

Soranus of Ephesus. *Diseases of Women*. Translated by H. Lueneburg. Munich: J. H. Lehmann, 1894.

Srinivasan, V., et al. "Therapeutic Actions of Melatonin in Cancer: Possible Mechanisms." *Integrative Cancer Therapies* 7, no. 3 (September 2008): 189–203.

Stamets, Paul. *Mycelium Running*. Berkeley, CA: Ten Speed Press, 2005.

Stevens, Richard G. "Artificial Lighting in the Industrialized World: Circadian Disruption and Breast Cancer." *Cancer Causes and Control* 17, no. 4 (May 2006): 501–507.

Stini, William A. "Bone Loss, Fracture Histories, and Body Composition." In *Bone Loss and Osteoporosis: An Anthropological Perspective*, edited by Sabrina C. Agarwal and Sam D. Stout. New York: Kluwer Academic/Plenum Press, 2003.

Stolley, Paul D., and Tamar Lasky. *Investigating Disease Patterns: The Science of Epidemiology*. New York: Scientific American Library, 1995.

Studzinski, G. P., and D. C. Moore. "Sunlight—Can It Prevent as Well as Cause Cancer?" *Cancer Research* 55, no. 18 (1995): 4014–22.

Stumph, W. E. "Vitamin D and the Digestive System," *European Journal of Drug Metabolism and Pharmacokinetics* 33, no. 2 (April/June 2008): 85–100.

"Sun Worship." *Columbia Encyclopedia*. 6th ed. New York: Columbia University Press, 2001.

"Symphysiotomy." *Managing Complications in Pregnancy and Childbirth: A Guide for Midwives and Doctors*. Department of Reproductive Health and Research, World Health Organization. 2002. http://www.who.int/reproductive-health/impac/ (accessed October 21, 2008).

Tangpricha, V., A. Turner, C. Spina, S. Decastro, T. C. Chen, and M. F. Holick. "Tanning Is Associated with Optimal Vitamin D Status (Serum 25-Hydroxyvitamin D

Concentration) and Higher Bone Mineral Density." *American Journal of Clinical Nutrition* 80, no. 6 (December 2004): 1645–49.

Tanko, L. B., Y. Z. Bagger, and C. Christiansen. "Low Bone Mineral Density in the Hip as a Marker of Advanced Atherosclerosis in Elderly Women." *Calcified Tissue International* 73, no. 1 (July 2003): 15–20.

Tanner, J. T., J. Smith, P. Defibaugh, et al. "Survey of Vitamin Content of Fortified Milk." *Journal of the Association of Official Analysis of Chemistry* 71 (1988): 607–10.

Teichmann, Anja, et al. "Sterol and Vitamin D2 Concentrations in Cultivated and Wild Grown Mushrooms: Effects of UV Irradiation." *Food Science and Technology* 40, no. 5 (June 2007): 815–22.

Thacher, T. D., P. R. Fischer, J. M. Pettifor, J. O. Lawson, C. O. Isichei, J. C. Reding, and G. M. Chan. "A Comparison of Calcium, Vitamin D, or Both for Nutritional Rickets in Nigerian Children." *New England Journal of Medicine* 341, no. 8 (August 1999): 563–68.

Tortora, Gerard J., and Sandra Reynolds Grabowski. *Introduction to the Human Body.* 5th edition. New York: John Wiley and Sons, 2001.

Ulett, G. "Geographic Distribution of Multiple Sclerosis." *Diseases of the Nervous System* 9 (1948): 342–46.

Van de Ven, W. S. "Mercury and Selenium in Cod-Liver Oil." *Clinical Toxicology* 12 no. 5 (1978): 579–81.

Vasquez, Alex, Gilbert Manso, and John Cannell. "The Clinical Importance of Vitamin D (Cholecalciferol): A Paradigm Shift with Implications for All Healthcare Providers." *Alternative Therapies* 10, no. 5 (September/October 2004): 28–36.

Vieth, Reinhold. "Effects of Vitamin D on Bone and Natural Selection of Skin Color: How Much Vitamin D Nutrition Are We Talking About?" In *Bone Loss and Osteoporosis: An Anthropological Perspective*, edited by Sabrina C. Agarwal and Sam D. Stout. New York: Kluwer Academic/Plenum Publishers, 2003.

———. "The Pharmacology of Vitamin D, Including Fortification Strategies." In *Vitamin D*, 2nd ed., edited by D. Feldman, F. H. Glorieux, J. W. Pike. San Diego: Academic Press, 1997.

———. "Vitamin D Supplementation, 25-Hydroxyvitamin D Concentrations, and Safety." *American Journal of Clinical Nutrition* 69, no. 5 (May 1999): 842–56.

———. "Why 'Vitamin D' Is Not a Hormone, and Not a Synonym for 1,25-Dihydroxy-vitamin D, Its Analogs or Deltanoids." *Journal of Steroid Biochemistry and Molecular Biology* 89–90 (2004): 571–73.

"Vitamin D Rights Bought for Bread." *New York Times*, March 10, 1931, 21: 6.

Vobecky, J. S., J. Vobecky, and L. Normand. "Risk and Benefit of Low Fat Intake in Childhood." *Annals of Nutrition and Metabolism* 39, no. 2 (1995): 124–33.

Waddell, J. "The Provitamin D of Cholesterol." *Journal of Biological Chemistry* 105 (July 1934): 711–39.

Walker, D. Carey, Soo-Voon Len, and Brita Sheehan. "Development and Evaluation of a Reflective Solar Disinfection Pouch for Treatment of Drinking Water." *Applied Environmental Microbiology* 70, no. 4 (April 2004): 2545–50.

Walsh, Bryan. "Beijing Smog Cleanup: Has It Worked?" *Time*, August 15, 2008. http://www.time.com/time/health/article/0,8599,1833371,00.htm (accessed October 18, 2008).

Weaver-Missick, Tara. "Boning Up on Navajo Food Habits." *Agricultural Research* (June 2001). http://www.ars.usda.gov/is/AR/archive/jun01/food0601.htm?pf=1 (accessed October 22, 2008).

Webb A. R., and M. F. Holick. "The Role of Sunlight in the Cutaneous Production of Vitamin D_3." *Annual Reviews in Nutrition* 8 (1988): 375–99.

Weiner, S. R. "Growing Pains." *American Family Physician* 27, no. 1 (January 1983): 189–91.

Wells, Spencer. *The Journey of Man.* New York: Random House, 2002.

Whiting, S. J., and M. S. Calvo. "Dietary Recommendations for Vitamin D: A Critical Need for Functional End Points to Establish an Estimated Average Requirement." *Journal of Nutrition* 135, no. 2 (February 2005): 304–309.

Wild, Martin Hans Gilgen, Andreas Roesch, Atsumu Ohmura, Charles N. Long, Ellsworth G. Dutton, Bruce Forgan, Ain Kallis, Viivi Russak, and Anatoly Tsvetkov. "From Dimming to Brightening: Decadal Changes in Solar Radiation at Earth's Surface." *Science* 308, no. 5723 (May 6, 2005): 847–50.

Wilhelm, Steven W., Markus G. Weinbauer, Curtis A. Suttle, and Wade H. Jeffrey. "The Role of Sunlight in the Removal and Repair of Viruses in the Sea." *Limnologyand Oceanography* 43, no. 4 (1998): 586–92.

Wincherts, I. S., N. M. van Schoor, et al. *Journal of Clinical Endocrine Metabolism* 92, no. 6 (June 2007): 2058–65.

Wolf, George, and Kenneth J. Carpenter. "Early Research into the Vitamins: The Work of Wilhelm Stepp." *Journal of Nutrition* 127 (July 1997): 1255–59.

Womack, K., Eric Russell T. Hill, Terri A. Muller, and Rita R. Colwell. "Effects of Sunlight on Bacteriophage Viability and Structure." *Applied and Environmental Microbiology* 62, no. 4 (April 1996): 1336–41.

Yang, Chun-Yuh, Hui-Fen Chiu, Chi-Ching Chang, Trong-Neng Wu, and Fung-ChangSung. "Association of Very Low Birth Weight with Calcium Levels in Drink-ingWater." *Environmental Research* 89 (2002): 189–94.

Zemel, Michael B., et al. "Regulation of Adiposity by Dietary Calcium." *FASEBJournal* 14 (2000): 1132–38.

Zittermann, A. "Vitamin D in Preventive Medicine: Are We Ignoring the Evi-dence?"*British Journal of Nutrition* 89, no. 5 (May 2003): 552–72.

Zubrow, Ezra. "The Demographic Modeling of Neanderthal Extinction." In *The Human Revolution: Behavioural and Biological Perspectives on the Origin of Modern Humans*, vol. 1. Edited by P. Mellars and C. B. Stringer. Edinburgh: Edinburgh University Press.

INDEX